50p

GW01162042

Biomarkers of dietary exposure

The term 'biomarker' has become increasingly popular in nutritional epidemiology in recent years. Biomarkers may provide a more valid and precise assessment of intake than dietary methods, especially for nutrients that vary widely in concentration within individual foods. However, for several important nutrients no feasible biomarker is available, and for others no biological measurements have been identified and validated yet. Despite the conceptual attractiveness, the application of biomarkers in nutritional epidemiology is confronted with important questions. Regarding the study hypothesis, it is important to distinguish between markers of exposure (the hypothesized causal factor), markers of disease (the endpoint affected), and markers of susceptibility (individual modifying factors). For each of these, one should consider sensitivity and specificity of the measurement; biological relevance in disease etiology; and collection, storage and laboratory analysis of the biological specimen.

The aim of the 3rd Meeting on Nutritional Epidemiology on 'Biomarkers of Dietary Exposure' held in 1991 in Rotterdam, The Netherlands is to contribute to a better understanding and broader application of biomarkers in future epidemiologic research on diet and disease.

These proceedings will provide you with an overview and perspective of the role of biomarkers, with the main emphasis on indicators of dietary exposure. Since there is great potential in epidemiologic research for the use of biomarkers as intermediate endpoints as well as markers of individual susceptibility for disease, these issues will also be addressed. Furthermore, the workshops on 'Energy', 'Fatty Acids', 'Selenium', and 'Antioxidants and Minor Food Constituents' are a reflection of current experiences in biomarker research. Finally, the presented abstracts and workshop reports, summarizing new developments and research priorities, are included in this book.

PROCEEDINGS OF THE 3rd MEETING
ON NUTRITIONAL EPIDEMIOLOGY

Biomarkers of dietary exposure

Edited by
Frans J Kok
Pieter van 't Veer

SMITH-GORDON
NISHIMURA

Smith-Gordon and Company Limited
Number 1, 16 Gunter Grove, London SW10 0UJ, Tel: 071 351 7042

Nishimura Company Limited
1–754–39 Asahimachi-Dori, Niigata-Shi 951, Japan

First published in Great Britain 1991.

British Library Cataloguing in Publication Data applied for

ISBN: 1-85463-071-7

Typeset by Reachword Limited, Sudbrooke, Lincoln.
Printed and bound in Great Britain by
Whitstable Litho Printers Ltd, Whitstable, Kent.

Contents

Preface

FRANS J KOK
Epidemiology Section, TNO Toxicology and Nutrition Institute, Zeist, The Netherlands

The term 'biomarker' has become increasingly popular in nutritional epidemiology in recent years. Biomarkers may provide a more valid and precise assessment of intake than dietary methods, especially for nutrients that vary widely in concentration within individual foods.

However, for several important nutrients no feasible biomarker is available, and for others no biological measurements have been identified and validated yet.

Despite the conceptual attractiveness, the application of biomarkers in nutritional epidemiology is confronted with important questions. Regarding the study hypothesis, it is important to distinguish between markers of exposure (the hypothesized causal factor), markers of disease (the endpoint affected), and markers of susceptibility (individual modifying factors). For each of these, one should consider sensitivity and specificity of the measurement; biological relevance in disease etiology; and collection, storage and laboratory analysis of the biological specimen.

The aim of the 3rd Meeting on Nutritional Epidemiology on 'Biomarkers of Dietary Exposure' held in 1991 in Rotterdam, The Netherlands is to contribute to a better understanding and broader application of biomarkers in future epidemiologic research on diet and disease.

These proceedings will provide you with an overview and perspective of the role of biomarkers, with the main emphasis on indicators of dietary exposure (Chapters 1–5). Since there is great potential in epidemiologic research for the use of biomarkers as intermediate endpoints as well as markers of individual susceptibility for disease, these issues will also be addressed (Chapters 6–8). Furthermore, the workshops on 'Energy', 'Fatty Acids', 'Selenium', and 'Antioxidants and Minor Food Constituents' (Chapters 9–12) are a reflection of current experiences in biomarker research. Finally, the presented abstracts and workshop reports, summarizing new developments and research priorities, are included in this book.

The 3rd Meeting on Nutritional Epidemiology follows two successful meetings in Berlin, one in 1988 on 'Epidemiology, Nutrition and Health' and the other in 1989 on 'The Diet History Method'.

This meeting on 'Biomarkers of dietary exposure' follows as a logical extension of these topics. This time, it has been organized by the TNO Toxicology and Nutrition Institute, Zeist, The Netherlands, in close cooperation with the WHO Collaborating Center for Nutritional Epidemiology in Berlin and the WHO Nutrition Unit in Copenhagen.

I am grateful to the members of the International Scientific Committee (Drs. Kohlmeier, Helsing, Huttunen, Hermus) and the National Committee

(Drs. Grobbee, Kromhout, van 't Veer), and to Ms. Flora de Vrijer and Ms. Hanny Leezer for the work done to make this meeting both interesting and pleasant to all participants.

The 3rd Meeting on Nutritional Epidemiology was sponsored by:
— Ministry of Welfare, Public Health and Cultural Affairs
— TNO Toxicology and Nutrition Institute
— Dairy Foundation on Nutrition and Health
— Unilever Research Laboratory

1

The use of biomarkers in nutritional epidemiology

WALTER C. WILLETT

Departments of Epidemiology and Nutrition, Harvard School of Public Health, Boston, USA

Introduction

The term biomarker has been used to describe measurements in the sequence of events leading from exposure, in this case diet, to disease[1]. At each step, persons may differ in susceptibility, thus a biomarker may also refer to an indicator of susceptibility. In the spirit of this conference, however, I will focus on biomarkers of diet.

The use of biomarkers is not new, although they have traditionally been referred to as indicators of nutritional status[2]. However, nutritional epidemiologists usually have a somewhat different perspective than traditional nutritionists. It is my perception that nutritionists have usually considered a measure of nutritional status, such as a biochemical measurement of blood or tissue to be of ultimate interest. In other words, once such a measure is available, one would have little interest in diet. However, dietary intake and nutritional status are really two different variables; both are inherently interesting in their own right. As epidemiologists we are often primarily interested in dietary intake and its relation to risk of disease because, from a public health standpoint, intake can be directly manipulated or altered through policy or individual behavioural changes. Nutritional status may be highly useful, even when not reflective of intake, simply because it is a

Biomarkers of dietary exposure. Ed. F. J. Kok & P. van 't Veer.

good predictor of disease. Serum cholesterol is a classical example. Serum cholesterol is a good predictor of coronary heart disease even though it is a poor indicator of dietary cholesterol. Thus, measuring serum cholesterol is minimally informative regarding the influence of dietary cholesterol on disease. Much confusion has arisen out of failure to distinguish between the use of a biochemical measure as a variable of direct interest or as an indicator of intake. Conceptual clarity is critical regarding the variable of interest. Sometimes the biomarker and dietary intake may be highly correlated, but at other times they may convey highly independent information.

Advantages of biomarkers of diet

Many reasons exist to be interested in biomarkers of diet. Biomarkers are said to be objective, which is particularly important in monitoring compliance in intervention studies. In virtually every intervention study in which self-reported compliance was compared with a biochemical measure of compliance, the former resulted in a too optimistic view. Biomarkers are sometimes said to be inexpensive. This may be true for a single nutrient, but they are usually costly if more than a few nutrients are measured. A fundamental advantage of biomarkers is that they are not dependent on knowledge of food composition or source. This is particularly valuable for contaminants, effects due to the processing of foods (such as isomerization of fatty acids), or certain micronutrients. The classical example is selenium, which can vary several orders of magnitude in different specimens of the same food, depending on where the food was produced. In such cases, biomarkers may play a unique role in assessing intake.

Another major advantage of biomarkers is that they can be available in retrospect. For example, epidemiologists have utilized frozen blood specimens collected many years before to conduct biochemical analyses. Using such an approach, questions can be addressed that were not conceived at the beginning of the study.

Biomarkers also can account for individual differences in bioavailability, absorption and metabolism. This can be both an advantage or disadvantage depending on whether intake or nutritional status is of interest.

Application of biomarkers of diet in nutritional epidemiology

In considering the use of biomarkers, several questions should be considered. Most fundamentally, is whether measure is sensitive to intake. Serum cholesterol and retinol are examples of common biochemical measures that are not very sensitive to intake. In contrast, serum carotenoids and vitamin E are quite responsive to diet so that blood levels are fairly sensitive indicator of intake.

How do we know whether a nutritional biomarker is sensitive to intake? Several types of studies can be informative. One approach is a cross-sectional study. For example, we have compared nail levels of selenium among countries where intakes were known to be substantially different[5]. In this cross-sectional analysis, a strong geographic correlation between nail selenium level and selenium intake was seen. This provided good evidence that the nail levels were sensitive to intake.

Small scale feeding studies to determine the response of the measure to intake can be informative; Dr. Katan will provide good examples of this approach. Often, the response of the tissue or blood nutrient level is non-linear in relation to intake. Thus, the question of whether the measure is sensitive to intake depends on the range of nutrient intake within the population to be studied. For example, when vitamin A intake is high, the biochemical marker may appear insensitive to intake. For this reason, serum retinol is not a good indicator of vitamin A intake in most developed countries. However, in many developing countries the intakes are very low, so that serum retinol may provide some information about vitamin A intake. Therefore, an evaluation of a biomarker of intake should be done in the context of the population for which the marker will be used.

Another approach is to compare a biomarker with intake measured directly. An example is provided by Longnecker and by Swanson[6] who evaluated several biomarkers of selenium intake. 44 adults were studied in South Dakota, an area where selenium intake is high and variable among persons. Selenium intake was measured directly by collecting replicate meals for these 44 people for 8 days over a one year period. The replicate meals for each day were blended and aliquoted to measure directly the selenium intake. Selenium measures of serum, blood and toenails were also obtained. These specimens provided the opportunity to examine the relative validity of these different methods for measuring selenium intake. The specimens also, incidentally, provided information about the best way of expressing selenium intake, as assessed by correlation with the biochemical measure. Not surprisingly, there was a better correlation with the tissue measures using intake expressed as intake per kilogram body weight than when using absolute intake. We also found that the correlations are very similar, on the order of 0.60, for the three different tissue measures, providing evidence that serum, whole blood, and toenails all provide relatively good measures of selenium intake.

A second consideration in evaluating a biomarker is the technical measurement error. An assessment of laboratory reproducibility is critical. Most of us as epidemiologists are collaborating with laboratory investigators who are doing the actual biochemical measurements. Laboratories should monitor and report their level of reproducibility themselves. However, in virtually every instance that we have examined, the reported lab coefficient of variation has been lower than the coefficient of variation found when we sent blind, split samples. For this reason, every laboratory collaboration should be preceded by sending blind split samples to estimate the technical error, as reflected by the within-person coefficient of variation. This is a most crucial issue from an epidemiologic standpoint. Obviously, it is desirable that the laboratory is calibrated against an external source, perhaps by participating in standardization programs. It is more difficult for an epidemiologist to evaluate systematic error of this type, but it is also less important in terms of estimating associations with disease.

The rapidity of response in the biochemical measure to dietary change is also important to an epidemiologist. In general, we want measures that are time-integrating, reflecting longer-term intake rather than intake over just a day or a few days. The degree to which a measure is time-integrating is a complicated function of several factors, including the variation of intake from day to day and the half-life of the biochemical measure. If a person eats exactly the same diet from one day to the next, it only would be necessary that the biochemical measure reflected diet over a period of a day or two. Unfortunately, most dietary factors vary greatly day-to-day, so that measures of intake that integrate over many days are highly advantageous. Because time integration is a complicated function of variation in intake and kinetics of the biomarker, collecting data on the half-life of the measure and detailed measures variation in dietary intake provide an arduous evaluation of whether or not a biochemical measure is adequate. A simple and straightforward way is to determine the reproducibility of the biochemical measure over time among individuals within the population to be studied. If the measure is reasonably reproducible over time, then it will be adequate in terms of time-integration.

In evaluating reproducibility, several questions arise. First, how long an interval of time should be evaluated? This obviously depends on the hypotheses to be addressed, but generally one should have at least two measures over an interval of months or years. For example, in a recent paper examining selenium levels in nails in relation to risk of breast cancer, we found a complete lack of association[3]. Having a subsample of nails collected six years apart in which a correlation of 0.60 over that period of time was seen substantially increased the credibility of the null finding. Without the reproducibility study, the possibility that of no consistency in selenium intake over time would have been difficult to dismiss. How high does the reproducibility correlation need to be? No clear cut-off exists; but some sense for an acceptable degree of correlation can be appreciated by considering the effects of various validity correlations (the correlation between the surrogate measure of intake and true intake) on observable relative risks[2]. For example, a validity correlation of 0.60 or 0.65 reduces the true excess relative risk (RR-1) by about half. This is a level of attenuation that we can live with in most epidemiologic studies, although this means we need a sample size approximately four-fold larger than if no error existed. The implication for reproducibility is that the square root of the reproducibility correlation is the validity correlation if error is only random within-persons. For example, if the correlation between two measures of blood pressure is 0.50, then the correlation between a single measure of blood pressure (validity correlation) and the average of a large number of measures of blood pressure would be the square root of 0.50, or about 0.70. This will be generally acceptable as a validity correlation. Considered in this way, we can probably tolerate reproducibility correlations down to, perhaps, 0.40 or so. Certainly we would prefer reproducibility correlations higher than 0.40, but this may not always be possible. In evaluating a biomarker, other extraneous factors that influence the levels should also be identified. Controlling those factors in the data analysis can reduce extraneous variation, and will then provide more precise estimates of validity.

Biomarkers available to nutritional epidemiologists

Biomarkers are presently available for many of the vitamins, a few minerals, specific fatty acids (as a percent of fatty acid intake), total protein intake, and energy (as expenditure). These are discussed elsewhere in detail[2]. However, for many dietary factors, biomarkers are either inadequate or unavailable. Unfortunately, those for which biomarkers are not available includes many of the variables in which we are most interested, such as for intakes of carbohydrates, total fat, absolute intake of fatty acids, and cholesterol.

Epidemiologic applications of biomarkers

As mentioned earlier, the assessment of compliance in trials will be an important application of biomarkers. However, such usage may often be limited by feasibility. Ultimately, we would like to apply biomarkers to case-control and cohort studies. Biomarkers may, nevertheless, be extremely valuable in validation studies. Used in this manner, biomarkers can provide insight regarding the interpretation of epidemiologic data, and in assessing the validity of our dietary intake methods.

As an example, Hunter et al., measured subcutaneous fatty acid levels in 118 men[4]. In these same men, dietary intake was measured by food frequency questionnaire and two one-week dietary records. For polyunsaturated fat intake expressed as absolute intake, the correlation with the subcutaneous adipose was very low. In contrast, expressed as percent fatty acids, the correlations were much higher (about 0.50). This provided rather direct evidence that expressing polyunsaturated fat consumption as absolute intake is not optimal with respect to biological relevance. This small study also provided important evidence that we are reasonably able to measure intake of polyunsaturated fat by either the food frequency questionnaire or the diet record. This validation study also provided estimates of the relative validity of the food frequency questionnaire and the 14 days of diet recording; because the correlations of two methods with adipose were very similar, their errors are likely to be of similar magnitude. In this same validation study, eicosapentanoic acid assessed by the food frequency questionnaire was also correlated with the same fatty acid in adipose. This is important information, because it means that our measure of intake from the questionnaire will be reasonably valid. Because such questionnaire data are available for about 250,000 people who are being followed (far too many to directly sample adipose), we will be capable of learning about the health effects of marine oils.

The advantage of having more than two measures of intake is further illustrated by saturated fat in the same study. For saturated fat, we observed only a weak correlation between both dietary assessment methods and the adipose, all expressed as a percent of total fatty acids. If we only had the food frequency questionnaire and the adipose, it would be hard to know which was wrong because the correlation was very weak. However, the two independent dietary methods were strongly correlated, and both correlated poorly with the adipose thus the most likely explanation is that the adipose is not a good measure of saturated fat intake. This also emphasizes one of the fundamental limitations of subcutaneous adipose measurements: we can only measure fatty acids as a percent of total fatty acids. Because saturated fat, which is measured poorly, will be in the denominator when measuring other fatty acids, any specific fatty acid is also going to be measured imperfectly as a percent of fatty acids. Although biomarkers attract considerable enthusiasm, they will not solve problems of confounding and bias that can arise in epidemiologic studies. Biomarkers may be just as subject to these problems as dietary intake, measures.

Summary

To conclude, further evaluation of existing biomarkers in terms of validity and long-term reproducibility is required for their optimal use in nutritional epidemiology. We need creativity in developing additional methods, particularly those that focus on long-term intake, using approaches such as protein adducts or mineral levels in nails, or lipid soluble factors. It will be important to compare these methods with intake assessment measurements to determine the relative validity of various approaches. Ultimately, the best nutritional epidemiologic studies will used a combination of dietary intake methods and biological markers, because some dietary factors will be measured well by questionnaire, but others can be measured optimally, and perhaps only, by biochemical assessments.

References

1 Hulka BS, Wilcosky TC, Griffith JD. Biological Markers in Epidemiology Oxford University Press, New York, 1990.
2 Hunter D. Biochemical indicators of dietary intake. In Nutritional Epidemiology, WC Willett ed. Oxford University Press, New York, 1990.
3 Hunter DJ, Morris JS, Stampfer MJ, Colditz GA, Speizer FE, Willett WC. A prospective study of selenium status and breast cancer risk. JAMA 1990; 264:1128-31.
4 Hunter D, Rimm EB, Sacks F, et al. Measurement of fatty acid intakes by subcutaneous fat aspirate, food frequency questionnaire, and diet records. Am J Epidemiol (abstract) 1990;132:752.
5 Morris JS, Stampher MJ, Willett WC. Dietary selenium in humans, toenails as an indicator. Biol Trace Element Res 1983;5:529-37.
6 Swanson CA, Longnecker MP, Veillon C, et al. Relation of selenium intake, age, gender, and smoking to indices of selenium status of adults residing in a seleniferous area. Am J Clin Nutr 1991 (in press).

2

What you should know about your marker

LENORE KOHLMEIER

Federal Health Office, WHO Collaborating Centre for Nutritional Epidemiology, Berlin, Germany

Types of Biomarkers

Biomarkers have been defined broadly as "indicators signalling events in biologic systems or samples" and generally classified into markers of "exposure, effect or susceptibility"[4]. This definition suffices for biomarkers in toxicology and in nutritional research. In contrast to the use of biomarkers in the field of toxicology, research on biomarkers which can be used for various purposes in nutritional epidemiologic studies is still in an early stage of development. The exposure variable in this case is food or nutrient intake; the effect variables are the measurable responses resulting from exposure in combination with physiologic characteristics and metabolic status of the subject. It is conceptually clearer in nutritional epidemiology to characterize the range of potential of biomarkers into six groups:

Biomarkers of intake, status, disease susceptibility, metabolic effect, disease occurrence and of compliance. Their relationship is presented in Figure 1.

1. Markers of *intake* reflect food or nutrient consumption directly, which is the central exposure parameter in nutritional epidemiology. These include markers of nutrient intakes such as selenium or β-carotene and markers of food intake, such as fish consumption[3].

Biomarkers of dietary exposure. Ed. F. J. Kok & P. van 't Veer.

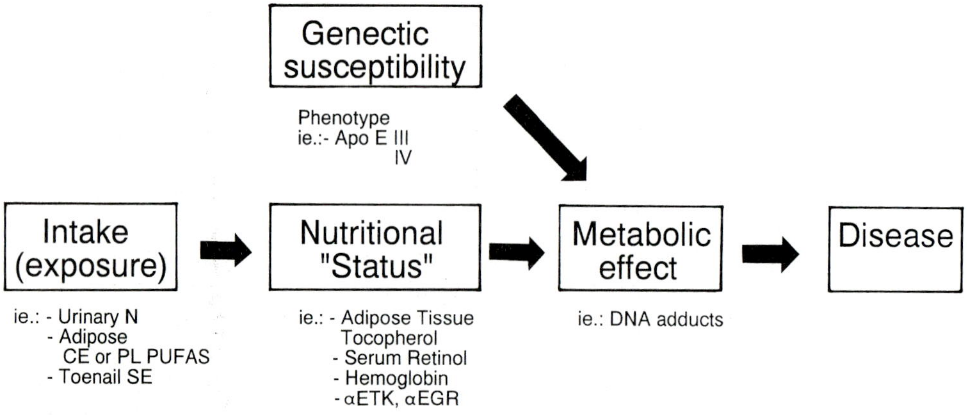

FIGURE 1. Pathway steps of interest and some corresponding biomarkers.

2. Unfortunately, nutritional *status* is often confused with intake although it is well known that the dietary intakes of many substances are only weakly related to storage or circulating levels. The status parameters which are generally measured tend to reflect more strongly the cascade of processes contained within the black box we call nutrition research[9] and includes the effects of adsorption, the transport of nutrients, their metabolism or storage, and their excretion. These measures include serum measurements of vitamins such as ascorbic acid, retinol, α-tocopherol or β-carotene.
3. The *susceptibility* of the subject to a given disease is a reflection of the genetic predisposition of the individual which may also be measured biologically. In the nutritional field, research on Apolipoprotein E pheno types promises a better understanding of the role of individual susceptibility to dietary responsiveness[5]. Furthermore, methods such as monoclonal antibodies, and more specifically, the polymerase chain reactions for the generation of DNA molecules swiftly, have opened new horizons and can be determined with relatively simple laboratory procedures in little material[8]. This use of DNA markers in research on the interaction between nutritional and genetic factors in the etiology of disease should reveal the levels of exposure needed to cause or protect from disease development in different individuals.
4. The combination of genetic susceptibility and nutritional status can result in measurable *metabolic effects* ranging from simple rate changes, to severe metabolic effects signalizing the preclinical stages of disease. The measurement of DNA adducts is an example of this group of biomarkers of preclinical disease development.
5. The classical parameters of interest in epidemiologic studies are exposures and the *occurrence of disease*. It is well known that diseases are not readily diagnosed in a timely and objective fashion. A diagnosis of disease requires a level of discomfort resulting in consultation with a

physician which differs between genders, between different age groups, and between individuals of the same sex and age and probably between countries and cultures. Objective measures of disease are sought after in epidemiologic research. Much of clinical chemistry is the science of identifying objective biomarkers of disease occurrence.

6. Independent of these pathways, biomarkers are being used to assess the validity of dietary assessment methods, of other biomarkers and of *compliance* with an intervention. These markers also play an important although separate role in nutritional epidemiology. Examples currently in use and contributing considerably to our knowledge include the use of doubly labelled water for energy expenditure calculations[11], PABA (para amino benzoic acid) for validation of 24 hour urine collections the use of lithium tagged salt to assess intake of discretionary sodium[14], or the use of urinary nitrogen to validate reported protein intakes[6]. Advances in measurement techniques, our understanding of factors influencing disease development and of genetic susceptibility to disease have promoted examination of the potential of biomarkers as affordable, objective and sensitive indicators for use in epidemiologic research.

Biomarkers of Intake

The focus of this scientific symposium is to provide an up-date on measurements which can be used as alternatives to the traditional dietary assessment methods which involve reporting, weighing, recalls, extensive interviews, estimation of portion sizes and in general subjective measures of assessing dietary intakes in an expensive and complex manner. A measure is being sought which will give the best possible indication of prior dietary intake over a broad period of time. The ideal relationship between dietary intake and its marker is linear, as in the theoretical association between vitamin E in plasma and vitamin E intake and illustrated in Figure 2. This relationship holds even at levels of supplementation 15 times that of the normal dietary intake levels[19].

Some relationships are however exponential, such as that between vitamin B2 intakes and riboflavin metabolites in urine (Figure 3). This mathematical problem, fortunately, can be solved by logarithmic transformation to achieve linearity. More difficult to deal with is a relationship such as that between vitamin C in plasma and ascorbic acid intakes, where a plateau effect is seen at high levels of intake (Figure 4). This makes the marker useless at high ranges of consumption. Another example of an unfavorable relationship is that between the intake and serum levels of retinol (Figure 5), making it practically unusable at any range of intake.

The biomarkers which allow direct assumptions of intake levels are still few and available for a limited number of nutrients. They include measures of long term intake of individuals as well as measures of change in individual intake.

Selenium in toenails is such a measure, which helps to classify individuals in terms of prior organic selenium consumption. It suffers however from

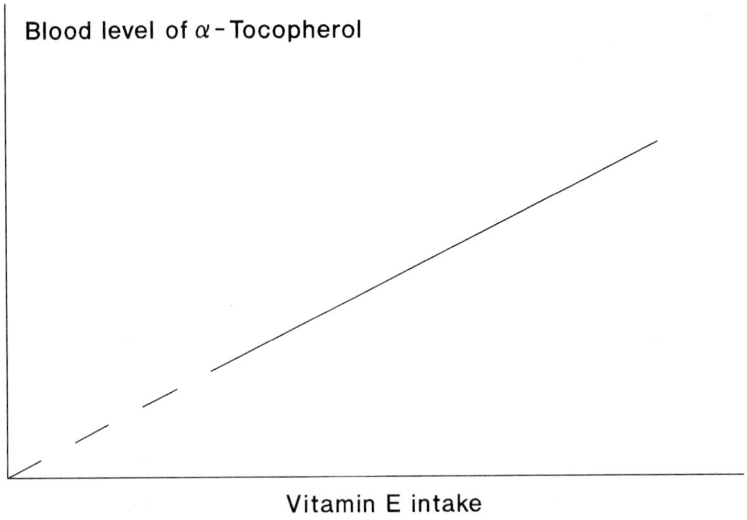

FIGURE 2. Relationship between vitamin E intake and blood level of alpha-tocopherol.

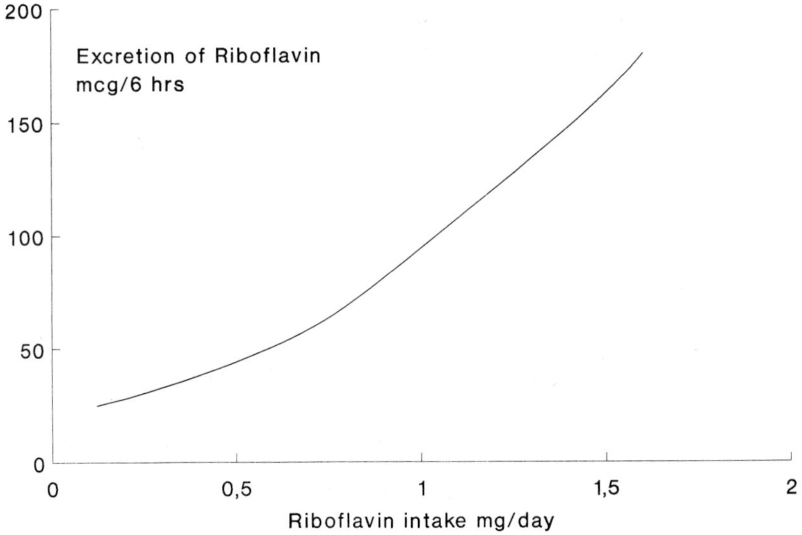

FIGURE 3. Relationship between vitamin B2 intake and excretion.

the fact that the intake of non-organic selenium is poorly reflected, and the denominator of the measure depends on rate of growth of toe nails[7,13]. External contamination (through selenium containing soaps and shampoo) need also be prevented.

The levels of specific polyunsaturated fatty acids such as linolenic and, or n-3 fatty acids, in adipose tissue, cholesterol-esters or phospholipids are also markers of intake which are currently the focus of intense interest among

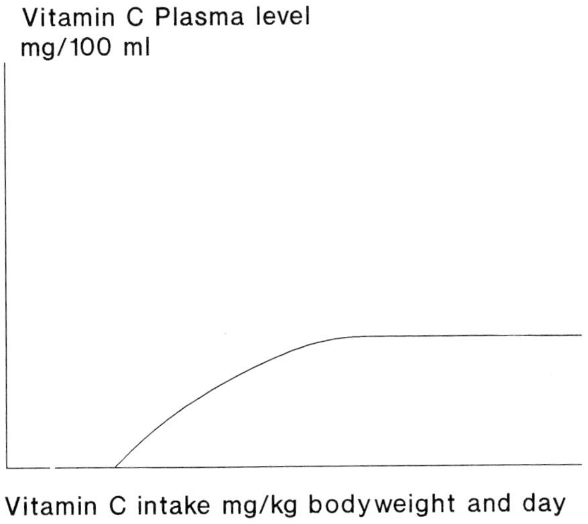

FIGURE 4. Relationship between vitamin C intake and vitamin C plasma level.

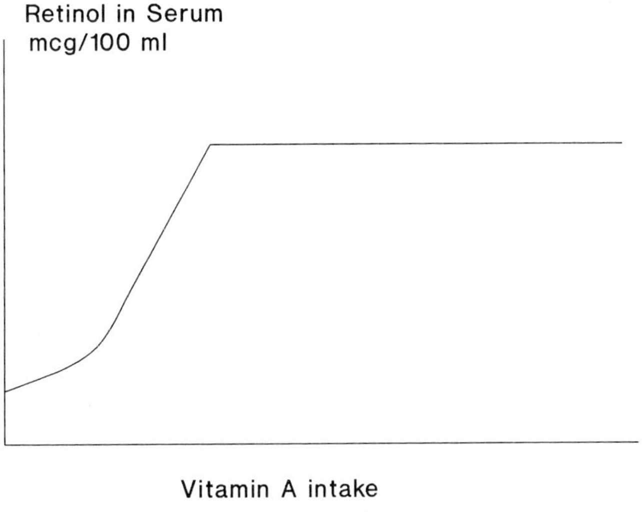

FIGURE 5. Relationship between vitamin A intake and retinol in serum.

nutrition researchers[1,2]. The long term intake of specific poly unsaturated fatty acids are well reflected in adipose tissue, whereas the short and intermediate changes in intakes are better reflected in more drastic changes in membrane and serum parameters.

In contrast to the vast amount of foods and nutrients in the diet which interest the nutritional epidemiologist, relatively few biomarkers of food or nutrient intake exist. Currently they seem to be limited to fatty acids, a few vitamins and some elements. These biomarkers reflect moderate and long term intakes.

Biomakers for the nutritional parameters which generally need at least to be controlled for in epidemiologic studies, such as alcohol intake, fat consumption and total energy intake do not exist.

And those markers which do exist are underresearched. For the appropriate and effective use of biomarkers of dietary intake, answers to a number of questions about the marker should be available. The fifteen important questions are presented below:

Fifteen Questions

1. What are you getting?

There are a number of substrates which can serve as potential media for biomarkers of exposures, ranging from exfoliated skin cells, blood, sweat or nails to bile, or urine. They are presented in Figure 6. In addition to the various body fluids and excretions, anthropometric parameters and measures of growth processes can serve as markers. When substrates are used, the tissue of interest should be specified and potential contamination by other natural tissues or external sources of the nutrient of interest, such as selenium in shampoo. Nail polish on toenails can alter the weight of the sample or provide undesired heavy metals considered. Toenails are subject to differences in rates of growth between persons, resulting in different samples reflecting different time periods in the past. In a fat aspiration, muscle or blood may affect the total weight and quality of the sample.

A second problem is determination of the denominator in calculations of concentration levels. Ear wax for example is theoretically attractive as a medium. It is a non invasively acquired lipid substrate for which however no theoretical basis for expecting similar concentrations between subjects exists since the mechanisms regulating production is poorly explored and-from which interindividual variation is high.

2. What are you losing?

Just as unexpected contaminants may be collected with a sample, undesired losses may affect the usefulness of the sample. This occurs to a degree in all handling of samples. The separation of serum, the isolation and preparation of fat tissue, incomplete 24 hour urine collections can all result in overestimation of the levels of the biomarker. The potential for losses during storage also need consideration, such as evaporations in frozen samples, which for example have led to the surprising result that the concentration of certain nutrients increases over time in stored samples.

3. Why is it there?

Particularly applicable to parameters of nutrient status, the question of why the nutrient is being found in the tissue sampled at the time in question is important in the interpretation of the results of the study. A circulating

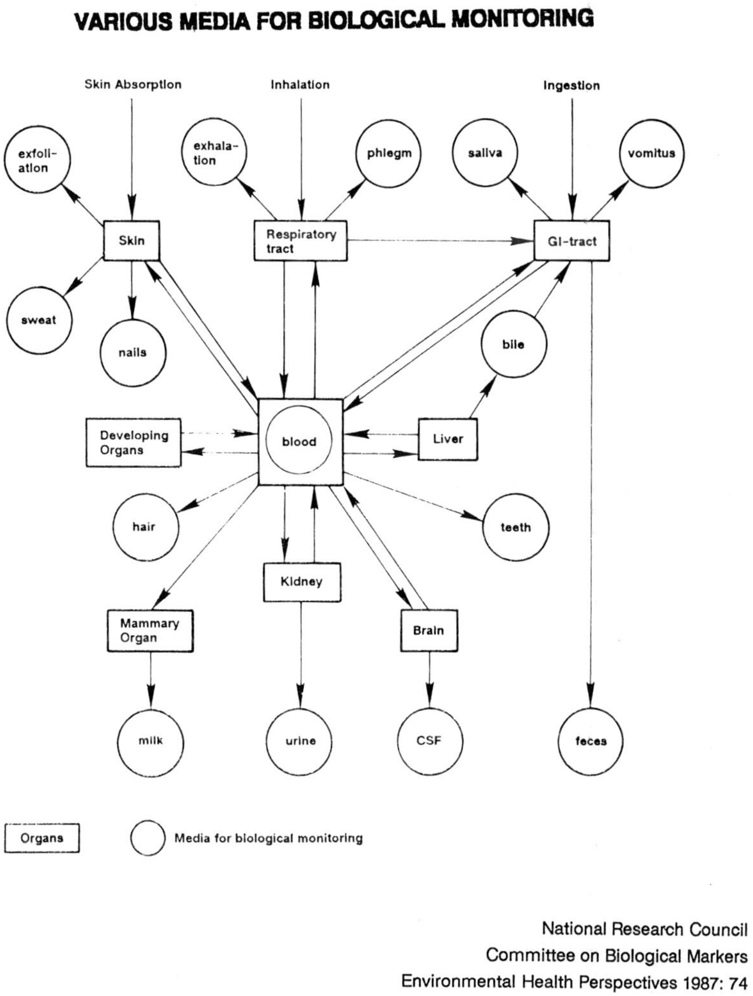

FIGURE 6. Various media for biological monitoring.

parameter may reflect sufficiency, storage, the availability of transport proteins or lipoproteins. It may be affected acutely by fever, or infection as is the case of serum iron levels or serum vitamin C levels.

4. When did it get there?

One tends to jump at the opportunity of using any biomarker which has proven to be a valid measure of intake, independent of the time frame of interest. Conceptual clarity on the time framework of the exposure measure of interest is needed, and a sober evaluation of whether the biomarker is a powerful enough indicator of intake at the exposure time of interest. The questions to ask are whether these are short term stores or long term deposits and what the half life of the nutrient in this tissue is.

5. What might have interfered with it getting there?
Inhibitors or promotors can affect the level of the marker in some individuals such that under similar intakes different intakes between individuals are seen. It is this type of differential bias which can make the biomarker useless as a measure of dietary exposure. The danger of this type of bias is that a result can be found which suggests a causal dietary role, but is in fact an artifact of the factors affecting a differential measure. For example, β-carotene levels may be lower due to smoking among cases in a study, not due to lower dietary intakes[16]. Or α-tocopherol levels in serum may be lower due to high fish consumption[15] rather than lower intakes.

6. Is this a storage, supply or excretion source?
The most readily available sample is most often used as a marker, and this is most frequently venous blood. Thus, supply and transport are the purpose of the presence of the biomarker, which need not, and does not in all cases reflect storage levels of nutrient. Vitamin C in serum, for example is measurable with some care and gives an impression of short term intakes (days). The concentrations of ascorbic acid in white blood cells reflects prior intakes going back weeks, and reflects more metabolic needs than transport. Circulating levels may be a function of transport proteins, as is the case with tocopherol levels in serum, which is carried on the low density lipoproteins. Tocopherol in general is contained largely in adipose tissue bulk lipid, where it is not generally exchangable[12]. Excretion amounts are also only a function of total stores in cases of steady state, not when metabolic activity levels are increased.

7. What has happened to the sample since sampling?
Although biomarkers are considered generally robust, during the process of handling and storage they are vulnerable to external contamination (iron), oxidation (ascorbic acid), temperature related changes. Possible evaporation has been mentioned earlier. These effects can result in falsely elevated or reduced measures as compared with the sample at the moment of collection.

8. What is the error range of the measurement?
There are many types and sources of measurement error; the most widely recognized is the laboratory measurement error. Validity, reproducibility and stability in measurement over time are components which are routinely measured as part of good laboratory practise through use of standards, blind samples, ring analyses and the running of control sera daily. The epidemiologist using the data should be familiar with the coefficients of variance in the sample at one point in time and over time, as well as the extent of deviation from the control measures, over the range of concentration relevant to the study.

9. What is the intraindividual variance of nutrient intake?
Before a good marker of intake of a given food or nutrient is found, conceptual clarity needs to exist about what is actually the exposure density over

time which is desired. Is one interested in the intake over the last days, the last months, the last years, or a given time interval from birth until the first development of disease? If the intraindividual intake is stable, any time frame can give a good assessment for the prior intake. If it is not stable, the time frame of observation needs to be wide enough to smooth out short term variation.

10. What is the intraindividual variance of the marker?
One often forgets that biomarkers also contain components of intraindividual variation. The rediscovery of this fact led to the widely hallowed statements of R. Peto that our estimations of risk in general are too low in epidemiologic research when adequate accounting for measurement error has not taken place. He uses the example of the effect of serum cholesterol levels on the risk of cardiovascular disease, and suggests that contrary to the reported result (LRC) that a 1% increase in cholesterol causes a 2% increase in the incidence of cardiovascular disease, it is actually a 3% increase which occurs, which is attenuated by measurement error (unpublished). The scientist should know how the measure of the marker varies from day to day and site to site within individuals.

Information on the within and betwen person variance of the marker will allow for the calculation the number of samples required to achieve the power sufficient to test adequately the hypothesis in question. A nice example of adjustment for this can be found in the calculations of Looker et al[12], in which they adjust for the prevalence estimates of iron deficiency based on the within and between person ratios, which varied from 0.03 for protoporphyrin to 2 for transferrin saturation. For β-carotene in plasma over a four week period ratios of 0.62 and for α-tocopherol 1.94 suggesting that as many as 3 to 8 repeat measures are needed to minimize attenuation[17].

11. Does the marker discriminate well at the levels of intake consumed?
Exposures which do not vary within a group can not be analyzed for risk by traditional epidemilogic means. In the same line, biomarkers which do not discriminate well within the range of interest are also not useful for epidemiologic studies on diets. So, for example, eicosapentanoic acid levels in erythrocytes was useful as a marker only for intakes above 150 mg/d[3].

12. What is the subject burden involved with sampling?
Realistic assessment of the burden of time, discomfort and risk of sampling, and the possible consequences for the subject of the sampling process as well as the potential benefits should be made. The current professional discussions on ethical standards for epidemiology may well result in the development of standards[10]. Currently, realistic appraisals of the consequences and risks of taking biopsies of muscle or fat for example are well advised.

13. What are the costs?
Not only the laboratory costs need to be calculated, but also the costs of

taking the sample (personnel and equipment), the cost of handling, storage and transport should not be underestimated. Transport often turns out to be the greatest cost in the use of fresh samples, and centralized labs.

14. When will the analyses be available?
The number of subjects generally enrolled in epidemiologic studies often surpasses the short term capabilities of laboratories for non-routine analytic measurements. It is advisable to know in advance when and in what form the analyses will be made available by the laboratory.

15. Are the results interpretable?
Often, due to enthusiasm, access to inexpensive laboratory technology, or scientific curiosity analyses are conducted which carry no underlying hypothesis or no power to test one. These uninterpretable results are ineffective and expensive. Furthermore they may lead one up a wrong alley. Currently, the literature on nutritional epidemiology is full of findings that nutritional biomarkers associate more strongly with disease occurrence than actual intake measures do. This may of course be due to lower measurement errors or biases in the measures. It may however also be due to the marker representing something other than dietary intake. For example, we still do not know what selenium in toenails means or what retinol in serum means in a nutritional sense. Only adequate knowledge and consideration of the above mentioned issues, and clarity about what the marker is, what it is influenced by and what it reflects allows for valid interpretation of the meaning of the result of the use of the marker for purposes of nutritional epidemiology. Lastly, one should be clear on whether it is a marker of diet, defect or of disease.

References

1 Allabriga A, Martinez A, Gallart-Catala A. Composition of subcutaneous fat depot in prematures in relationship with fat intake. Helv Paediat Acta 1972;27:91–8.
2 Beynen AC, Hermus RJJ, Hautvast JGAJ. A mathematical relationship between the fatty acid composition of the diet and that of the adipose tissue in man. Am J Clin Nutr 1980;33:81–5.
3 Brown AJ, Roberts DCK. Erythrocyte EPA as a marker for intake of fish and fish oil. Eur J Clin Nutr 1990;44:487–8.
4 Committee on Biological Markers of the National Research Council. Biological Markers in Environmental Health Research. Environ Health Persp 1987;74:3–9.
5 Eichner JE, Kuller LH, Ferrell RE, Meilahn EN, Kamboh MI. Phenotypic effects of apolipoprotein structural variation on lipid profiles. III. Contribution of apolipoprotein E phenotype to prediction of total cholesterol, apolipoprotein B, and low density lipoprotein cholesterol in the Healthy Women Study. Genet Epidemiol 1990;3:379–85.
6 Hultén B, Bengtsson C, Isaksson B. Some errors inherent in a longitudinal dietary survey revealed by the urine nitrogen test. Eur Ju Clin Nutr 1990;44:169–74.
7 Hunter DJ, Morris JS, Chute CG, Kushner E, Golditz GA, Stampfer MJ, Speizer FE, Willett WC. Predictors of selenium concentration in human, toenails. Am J Epidemiol 1990;132:114–22.
8 Khoury MJ, Beaty TH, Flanders WD. Epidemiologic approaches to the use of DNA markers in the search for disease susceptibility genes. Epidemiol Rev 1990;12:41–55.

9 Kohlmeier L, Helsing E. Analytical problems in nutritional epidemiology. In: Epidemiology, Nutrition and Health. Proceedings of the 1st Berlin Meeting on Nutritional Epidemiology. Smith-Gordon, London 1988;9–18.
10 Last JM. Association News. Guidelines on Ethics for Epidemiologists. Int J Epidemiol 1990;19:226–9.
11 Livingstone MBE, Prentice AM, Coward WA, Ceesay SM, Strain JJ, McKenna PG, Nevin GB, Barker ME, Hickey RJ. Simultaneous measurement of free-living energy expenditure by the doubly labeled water method and heart-rate monitoring. Am J Clin Nutr 1990;52:59–65.
12 Looker AC, Sempos CT, Liu K, Johnson CL, Gunter EW. Within-person variance in biochemical indicators of iron status: effects on prevalence estimates. Am J Clin Nutr 1990;52:541–7.
13 Salbe AD, Levander OA. Effect of various dietary factors on the deposition of selenium in the hair and nails of rats. J Nutr 1990;120:200–6.
14 Sanchez-Castillo CP, Seidell J, James WPT. A test of the validity of the lithium-marker technique for monitoring dietary sources of salt in man. Clin Sci 1987;72:87–94.
15 Schäfer L, Overad K. Subcutaneous adipose-tissue fatty acids and vitamin E in humans: relation to diet and sampling site. Am J Clin Nutr 1190;52:486–90.
16 Stryker WC, Kaplan LA, Stein EA, Stampfer MJ, Sober A, Willett WC. The relation of diet, cigarette smoking, and alcohol consumption to plasma β-carotene and α-tocopherol levels. Am J Epidemiol 1988;127:283–96.
17 Tangney CC, Shekelle RB, Raynor W, Gale M, Betz EP. Intra- and interindividual variation in measurements of β-carotene, retinol, and tocopherol in diet and plasma. Am J Clin Nutr 1987;45:764–9.
18 Traber MG, Kayden HJ. Tocopherol distribution and intra cellular localization in human adipose tissue. Am J Clin Nutr 1987;46:488–95.
19 Urbach C, Hickman K, Harris PL. Effect of individual vitamins A, C, E and carotene administered at high levels on their concentration in the blood. Exp Med Surg 1952;10:7–20.

3

Overview of biomarkers of dietary intake

FRANS J KOK and PIETER VAN 'T VEER

Epidemiology section, TNO Toxicology and Nutrition Institute, Zeist, The Netherlands

Introduction

In nutritional epidemiology the primary interest is in biomarkers, which adequately reflect nutrient intake. These exposure markers can be used in etiologic research either as an alternative or in addition to dietary questionnaires. Biomarkers may provide a more valid and precise assessment of intake than dietary methods, especially for nutrients that vary widely in concentration within individual foods or for nutrients from foods that cannot be assessed reliably. Despite the conceptual attractiveness, the application of biomarkers in nutritional epidemiology is confronted with important questions e.g., sensitivity and specificity of the measurement; biological relevance in disease etiology; and collection, storage and laboratory analysis of the biological specimen. In this paper we will concentrate on biologic, epidemiologic and laboratory aspects relevant in evaluating the usefulness of biological markers of dietary exposure.

Biomarkers may be defined as cellular, biochemical or molecular alterations that are measurable in biological media, such as human tissues, cells or fluids[4]. Next to 'markers of exposure', their is great potential in nutritional epidemiology for the use of 'markers of susceptibility' and 'markers of disease'. Susceptibility markers may be genetically determined or acquired through life. The ApoE phenotype is an example from the cardiovascular field. Subjects with this genetic trait are susceptible to hypercholesterolemia

Biomarkers of dietary exposure. Ed. F. J. Kok & P. van 't Veer.

and therefore have an increased risk to coronary heart disease. In stead of clinical disease as an endpoint, biomarkers of earlier stages in the disease process are preferable in etiologic research. These 'markers of disease', also called early endpoints, we find especially in cancer research. Examples are oncogene activation, bronchial dysplasia, and colon polyps. The different types of biomarkers have been used by many epidemiologists in their research[4]. Cardiovascular disease epidemiologists have focused on serum cholesterol, lipids and lipoprotein fractions with great success. This approach has increased our knowledge of the causes of atherosclerosis and myocardial infarction. In cancer epidemiology several cancer precursors are in use, and in the more basic nutrition sciences, biochemical indicators are applied to evaluate nutritional status and nutrient metabolism in individuals.

Framework for biomarkers

Figure 1 shows a framework for the use of biomarkers in epidemiologic research. It covers the whole spectrum from dietary intake to clinical disease occurrence. It is taken from the National Research Council's Committee on Biological Markers in Environmental Health[6]. Interestingly, biomarkers receive increasing attention in studies on the health effects of environmental and occupational exposures. Because of the focus of this meeting we will concentrate on the left side, biomarkers of dietary exposure. First the scheme in figure 1 is explained in more detail and some biological media for markers are considered.

The framework for the different types of biomarkers, is clarified by three examples: One for the well-known relation between smoking and lung cancer, the second for saturated fat intake and coronary heart disease, and the third for nutritional factors in breast cancer etiology (Table 1). Regarding exposure we distinguish internal and effective dose. The internal dose directly reflects the habit of smoking itself by assessment of a nicotine metabolite namely cotinine. This metabolite clearly acts as a marker of the habit of smoking with its associated detrimental exposures, rather than as a causally involved intermediate as such. The effective dose indicates the biologically relevant

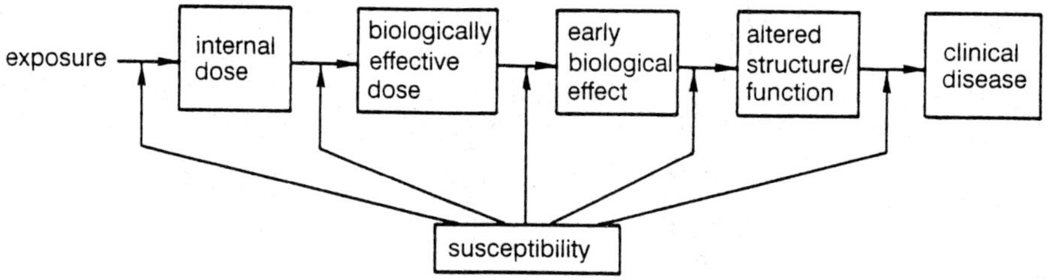

FIGURE 1. Framework for biological markers (examples in text). The markers represent a continuum and the classification may not always be distinct (From National Research Council: ref 6).

TABLE 1. Examples of biomarkers.

Biomarker	Exposure		
	Smoking	Saturated fat	Fat, Fiber
Internal dose	cotinine	LDL-cholesterol	(non-)nutrients
Effective dose	DNA-adducts	oxidized LDL	hormones
Early response	SCEs,	fatty streaks	oncogenes
Early endpoint	dysplasia	angina pectoris	hyperplasia
Clinical disease	lung cancer	myocardial infarction	breast cancer
Susceptibility	GST-μ	ApoE	fat distribution

interaction of the exposure with a critical subcellular target (DNA adducts in the smoking example). Regarding the biological response to exposure usually the hard endpoint (clinical disease) is chosen. However, earlier stages in the pathogenesis of the disease may be more relevant to the exposure of interest. Early endpoints (bronchial dysplasia in the smoking example) and early response markers such as Sister Chromatid Exchanges (SCE) in lymphocytes or micronuclei in sputum may even reflect a more crucial step very early in carcinogenesis. Finally, some subjects may be particularly susceptible to damage by cigarette smoke. For example, Van Poppel et al[11] observed increased SCEs in smokers who were genetically deficient in the enzyme glutathione transferase-μ.

The second example relates to the intake of saturated fat and risk of myocardial infarction. LDL-cholesterol and oxidized LDL may be considered as biomarkers of internal and effective dose for saturated fat intake. Fatty streaks and angina pectoris are manifestations of early response and early endpoint, respectively. ApoE phenotype is one possible genetic marker of susceptibility.

The last example is less specific, since feasible biomarkers for dietary factors related to breast cancer, such as fat and fiber intake, are lacking. Furthermore, the target tissue concentration of hormones is likely to be more relevant than the easily accessible plasma concentrations. Regarding disease biomarkers, attention might shift from overt clinical disease to oncogene activation or to early endpoints such as atypical hyperplasia or proliferative disease. With respect to susceptibility it could be conceived that the fat distribution (apple, pear) may be a promising biomarker of a specific hormonal phenotype.

Media for Biomarkers

The markers in Table 1 should be assessed in one of the many potentially available biological media (Figure 2). The following media are usually con-

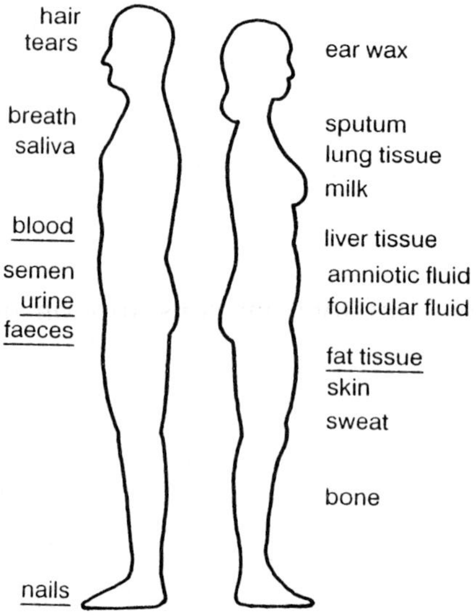

FIGURE 2. Media for biomarkers. Underlined media are commonly used in nutritional epidemiology (see text).

sidered as markers for dietary intake: blood (fatty acids, vitamins), urine (nitrogen, electrolytes), faeces (non-digestible fiber, bulk), nails (selenium, other trace elements), fat tissue (fatty acids, vitamins). Some of these are more feasible for epidemiologic studies among free living subjects (blood, nails, urine, fat tissue), while the use of some other media is necessarily restricted to a metabolic ward setting (faeces). Other media (e.g., bone and liver tissue) may be available only under clinical conditions.

Biomarkers of Dietary Exposure

Table 2 gives a simple listing of nutrients for which biomarkers do exist. Both for macronutrients, vitamins and minerals, valuable information on biomarkers can be derived from reviews by Hunter[5], Riboli[8], and Hebert and Miller[1]. For several important nutrients no feasible biomarkers are available, and for others no biomarkers have been identified and validated yet. For

TABLE 2. Biomarkers of dietary exposure.

Macronutrients	Vitamins	Minerals
protein	vit A, D, E, K	Se, Fe, Zn, Cu
fatty acids	carotenoids	Na, K, Ca, Mg
alcohol	vit B1, B2, B6	
energy	vit C, folic acid	

other nutrients, specific indicators of biological response may serve as markers of exposure (e.g. HDL-cholesterol for alcohol intake and LDL-cholesterol mainly for saturated fatty acids and partly for cholesterol intake).

For applications in epidemiology, however, the overview in Table 2 does not suffice because it does not take into account the actual performance of biomarkers in a practical research setting. For instance, if the interest is in type of fat, the table does not help us to choose between the fatty acid profile of serum cholesteryl esters or alternatively in aspirated adipose tissue. On the other hand, for total fat consumption no adequate longterm marker of intake is readily available. For the nutritional epidemiologist it is extremely important to know the criteria for evaluating the usefulness of a biomarker.

Evaluation criteria for use of biomarkers

Knowledge on biology, epidemiology and on laboratory aspects is relevant in evaluating the performance of a biomarker of dietary exposure. In Table 3 most of the important aspects are summarized. Of course, there are many interrelations between the different aspects. Nutrient metabolism affects the body pools of the biomarker and, therefore, it is relevant to the selection of the optimal biological medium, namely target or surrogate tissue.

For instance, the chemical form of selenium in toenails does not necessarily reflect the body pool relevant to carcinogenesis. Regarding biology, we have to take into account the physiological properties of the nutrient biomarker such as its metabolism, time integration and potential other determinants of the biomarker level. This should be supplemented with knowledge of pathogenesis, relating to the concepts of induction time and the disease stage affected by the exposure assessed by the biomarker. These biological issues have implications in designing nutritional epidemiologic research, for example is the purpose the validation of a questionnaire or the

TABLE 3. Relevant aspects of biomarkers.

Biology	*Physiology* Nutrient metabolism Time integration Other determinants	*Pathogenesis* Induction time Disease stage
Epidemiology	*Design* Validation vs etiology Prospective vs retrospective Single vs repeated measurements	*Feasibility* Target vs surrogate tissue Free living vs metabolic ward Invasiveness and acceptability Ethical considerations
Laboratory	*Sample analysis* Complexity sample preparation Precision and validity Sensitivity and specificity Destructive, non-destructive	*Pre-analytical stage* Collection, transport, storage Temperature, light, oxygen Aliquots for other analyses Internal and external references

elucidation of disease etiology. Additional epidemiologic issues include feasibility aspects such as invasiveness of procedures, willingness of participants and ethical considerations.

Laboratory aspects refer to such things as accuracy and precision of the biomarker measurement, sample-handling and costs of analysis. We will not evaluate all the nutrient biomarkers in Table 2, according to all the criteria mentioned in Table 3. Biomarkers of β-carotene and retinol are chosen to illustrate one or two of the aspects from biology, epidemiology and the laboratory.

Biology
Regarding biology, it is first important to consider nutrient metabolism. For example, in the left part of Figure 3, plasma retinol levels are low (vitamin A deficient population). The metabolic conversion of dietary β-carotene to retinol helps to restore plasma retinol levels, and thereby supplements the dietary retinol intake. A second issue relevant to biomarkers of dietary exposure is illustrated in the right part of the figure.

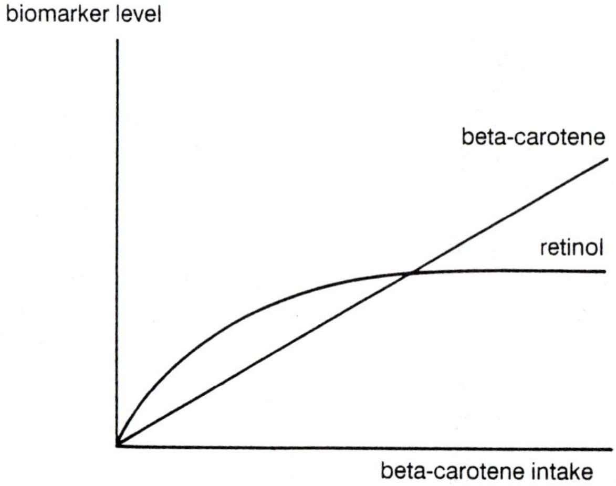

FIGURE 3. Nutrient metabolism and biomarker performance. Because of beta-carotene conversion, plasma retinol does reflect beta-carotene intake, but only at low intake levels in vitamin A deficient populations. Plasma beta-carotene is a biomarker of intake over a much wider range.

Here, plasma β-carotene levels are still determined by diet and can be used as biomarkers of intake. Plasma retinol, however, is no longer sensitive to dietary β-carotene. Finally, knowledge of pathogenesis is essential for the selection of a biomarker. Thus, β-carotene might play a dual role as both an antioxidant and as provitamin-A in carcinogenesis, while its role in atherogenesis may be restricted to its antioxidant properties.

Epidemiology
Some epidemiologic issues relevant to biomarkers can be illustrated using part of the results from a case-control study on β-carotene and breast cancer, published by Potischman[7]. In this study, the odds ratios in the highest to lowest quartile of plasma β-carotene were 1.0, 1.2, 1.8 and 3.2, respectively. No association, however, was seen for dietary β-carotene intake (Odds ratios for highest to lowest quartile 1.0, 1.5, 1.7, 1.3). Among other possibilities, these results might suggest that the lower β-carotene plasma levels in cases might be a consequence of the disease rather than a result of dietary intake. This inferential problem may not rise in a prospective study design, where blood samples are collected several years before clinical disease. An alternative explanation of the case-control results would be that the lower plasma levels may have arise from dietary habits, altered in the days or week before diagnosis. Such alterations may not have influenced the reported dietary habits yet, but they may have affected plasma levels already. A longterm biomarker of b-carotene in adipose tissue might have been less sensitive to such recent changes in dietary habits. In addition to etiologic studies, biomarkers also play an important role in the validation of dietary methods, while supplementation studies may learn us more about the biological properties of the exposures of interest.

Laboratory aspects
The major laboratory aspects for the evaluation of biomarkers are: sample collection, transport, storage and analysis. All these aspects may influence the validity and precision of the biomarker measurement in the laboratory. Here we will focus on precision of the measurements. Note that lack of precision will result in misclassification of exposure status and, consequently, to dilution of the exposure-disease associations. We illustrate two important points regarding precision. First, there may be quite a substantial difference in routine vs optimal precision of the measurements, indicated by the coefficient of variation (CV).

Optimal precision is usually achieved under strictly controlled laboratory conditions. Such conditions can usually not be maintained during the course of large-scale epidemiologic studies that involve many analysts, equipment and a long period of time. This is clearly seen for plasma retinol, assessed by HPLC. In routine vs optimal laboratorium conditions, the CV was 9.1% and 3.7%, respectively[9]. Second, the amount of sample-material collected may be of critical importance. Analysis of a large 1 ml sample can be conducted with considerably higher precision than a 5 l sample both in routine analysis (CV = 13.0%) as well as under optimal laboratory conditions (CV = 6.7%). In conclusion, one cannot simply use the coefficient of variation as such, but should consider the amount of material collected as well.

Early endpoint markers

So far, we have concentrated on the left side of Figure 1, namely exposure markers. For a complete picture, early endpoint markers and susceptibility markers need some attention as well.

In other chapters in the proceedings, these markers will be addressed in more detail (2,10). To illustrate the concept of early endpoints in nutritional epidemiology, we use data published by Hislop[3]. In this study, women in a screening program were diagnosed as having benign breast disease. Women with 'proliferative disease', a potential biological precursor of breast cancer, were considered to experience increased breast cancer risk. Among these women, the odds ratios for high intake of green vegetables (rich in β-carotene) and vitamin A supplements were 0.3 (frequent vs rare consumption) and 0.5 (users vs non-users), respectively. For women without 'proliferative disease', however, no association with these dietary exposures was observed (Corresponding odds ratios were 1.4 and 1.2, respectively). Thus, β-carotene and retinol are inversely associated with 'proliferative disease' in this study. By identifying the subgroup of women at increased breast cancer risk, the association with carotenoids and retinoids has become more pronounced. This association would have been much weaker or might not have been observed at all if benign breast disease was not further classified according to future breast cancer risk. Thus, failure to recognize relevant disease precursors, may leave biologically meaningful associations undetected.

Biomarkers of individual susceptibility

Now that we have discussed the range of biomarkers from dietary exposure to (early) endpoint, we are left with the biomarkers of individual susceptibility. Figure 4 depicts how disease risk is related to dietary exposure among

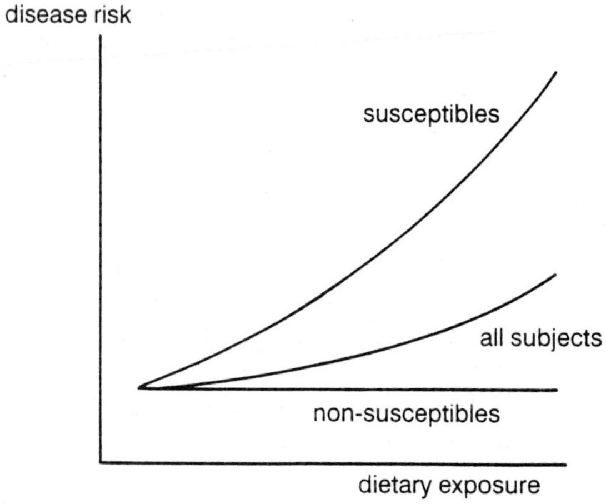

FIGURE 4. Biomarkers of susceptibility. Disease risk associated with dietary exposure will be highest in subjects with inherited or acquired susceptibility. Usually, susceptibility has to be ignored and some attenuated association is observed in epidemiologic research.

non-susceptible subjects compared to susceptibles. In this hypothetical example, non-susceptibles are not at increased risk at high exposure. This can be the case because the relevant harmful dietary factor is not absorbed, not transported to the target organ, the biological harm is efficiently repaired, or the detrimental substance is efficiently metabolized and excreted. This way there is an optimal defense of the body. If a subject has the right genetic constitution all these different metabolic conversions are favorably handled. If the subjects have the opposite genetic constitution, they will experience increased risk already at low dietary intake, and even more so at high exposure levels. In practice, we usually have to ignore the hereditary and acquired genetic constitution of individuals. Therefore, the association we observe in our studies is somewhere between the association for susceptibles and non-susceptibles (see the line in the middle). Its exact position depends on the proportion of both groups of subjects in the study population. It should be realized that the more genes involved in determining susceptibility, however, the more difficulties we will have to study their separate contribution to clinical disease.

Epilogue and conclusions

As we have seen above, biomarkers give useful additional insight in our research activities. There are several reservations, however, and we should not be over-enthusiastic. Note that we have used β-carotene only for qualitative illustration of some relevant issues, not for a quantitative evaluation of its performance using all the relevant criteria. It is questionable whether all biomarkers of dietary exposure (Table 2) could stand such a rigorous test. Furthermore, several nutrients simply lack biomarkers, and for others we may never be able to find adequate biomarkers, or we don't need them.

Finally, biomarkers are important to assess exposure to specific nutrients, but the dietary questionnaire may still be more adequate to characterize diet and take preventive action, either at the individual or at the population level.

Apart from these reservations, biomarkers hold clear promises for nutritional epidemiology, especially regarding methodology. They may help to improve precision, to reduce misclassification and thus to strengthen the diet-disease associations of interest. They may demonstrate effect modification and identify subgroups at particular risk, either because of their genetic constitution, or because of the stage of disease already developed. Finally, biomarkers may enhance the understanding of the mechanisms of disease occurrence, which is possible if biomarkers are themselves part of the causal link between exposure and disease.

In our daily research practice we will have various kinds of problems in the development, testing and use of biomarkers. The application of existing and new biomarkers of dietary exposure requires intense collaboration among epidemiologists, nutritionists, clinicians and laboratory researchers. Although this is not the place for elaboration on this topic, ethical considerations come into the picture when we are going to apply less common or more invasive methods for sampling biological media, or when genetic factors are of relevance. There is no need to say that the latter is not the simplest part of our job. A balanced view on the reservations and promises attached to biomarkers, however, will certainly help us to overcome these practical constraints.

References

1 Hebert JR, Miller DR. Methodologic considerations for investigating the diet-cancer link. Am J Clin Nutr 1988;47:1068–77.

2 Hemminki K, Mustonen R, Reunanen A, et al. Application of DNA adduct measurements for dietary studies. In: Biomarkers of dietary exposure, ed. FJ Kok and P van 't Veer 1991. Smith-Gordon, London pp. 59–66.

3 Hislop GT, Band PR, Deschamps M, et al. Diet and histologic types of benign breast disease defined by subsequent risk of breast cancer. Am J Epidemiol 1990;131:263–70.

4 Hulka BS, Wilcosky TC, Griffith JD. Biological markers in epidemiology. Oxford University Press, New York, 1990.

5 Hunter D. Biochemical indicators of dietary intake. In: Nutritional Epidemiology, ed. WC Willett. New York: Oxford University Press 1990:143–216.

6 National Research Council, Committee on Biological Markers. Biological markers in environmental health research. Environ Health Perspect 1987;74:3–9.

7 Potishman N, McCulloch CE, Byers T, et al. Breast cancer and dietary and plasma concentrations of carotenoids and vitamin A. Am J Clin Nutr 1990;52:909–15.

8 Riboli E, Rm H, Saracci R. Biological markers of diet. Cancer Surveys 1987;6:685–718.

9 Speek AJ. Vitamin analysis in body fluids and foodstuffs with high-performance liquid chromatography (Thesis). TNO Toxicology and Nutrition Institute, Zeist, Netherlands, 1989.

10 Tikkanen MJ. Biomarkers for the apolipoprotein B gene, a candidate gene for atherosclerosis. In: Biomarkers of dietary exposure, ed. FJ Kok and P van 't Veer 1991. Smith-Gordon, London pp. 67–73.

11 Van Poppel G, De Vogel N, Van Bladeren PJ, Kok FJ. DNA damage in heavy smokers favourably influenced by glutathione transferase phenotype. (Submitted).

4

Biological markers of dietary intake with emphasis on fatty acids

MARTIJN B KATAN, ANGÉLIQUE VAN BIRGELEN, JEAN P DESLYPERE[1], MARGRIET PENDERS and WIJA A VAN STAVEREN

Department of Human Nutrition, Wageningen Agricultural University, Wageningen, The Netherlands
[1]Department of Endocrinology and Hematology, State University Ghent, Ghent, Belgium

Summary

The level of certain polyunsaturated fatty acids in body fluids or tissues can be a valid indicator of their consumption in man. In 59 housewives studied over a 2.5 y period we found a correlation of 0.70 between the intake of linoleic acid, assessed as the mean of 19 24-h recalls, and the level in fat tissue[5]. In 58 adult men supplemented with fish oil capsules for a year, the rise of eicosapentaenoic acid levels in erythrocyte membranes was strongly and specifically related to the rise in intake. We conclude that epidemiological studies of the role of these fatty acids in health and disease could fruitfully employ these markers of dietary intake.

Introduction

The lack of accurate and reproducible methods for the assessment of nutrient intake is a major obstacle for research on the relation between diet and health. For that reason there is much interest in objective biochemical pa-

Biomarkers of dietary exposure. Ed. F. J. Kok & P. van 't Veer.

rameters that reflect dietary intake. The more successful markers developed hitherto (Bingham SA, this volume) are those for protein (via urinary nitrogen), energy (via the doubly-labelled water technique), sodium and potassium (urinary excretion), and markers for the intake of various fatty acids. The essential (n-6) polyunsaturated fatty acid linoleic acid has been studied most. The content of this fatty acid in various fractions reflects a moving average of the intake over preceding periods of time of various lengths.

Thus the linoleic acid content of cholesteryl esters in blood serum reflects the diet of the preceding weeks and that of erythrocyte membranes that of the preceding 2–3 months, while the linoleic acid content of microbiopsies of subcutaneous fat tissues faithfully reflects individual consumption over the preceding 1 to 3 years. All these parameters can now be measured routinely in epidemiological studies.

Recently we have turned our attention to markers for other fatty acids, including the (n-3)polyunsaturated fatty acids (w3-fatty acids) typically found in marine oils. Here we review some of our experience with linoleic acid in adipose tissue as a marker of long-term intake, and we present some preliminary data on the (n-3)polyunsaturates.

Methods and results

The study on linoleic acid in adipose tissue has been described in detail in reference[5]. Figure 1 presents the design. Briefly, 66 housewives living in the town of Renkum were each questioned about their dietary intake 19 times

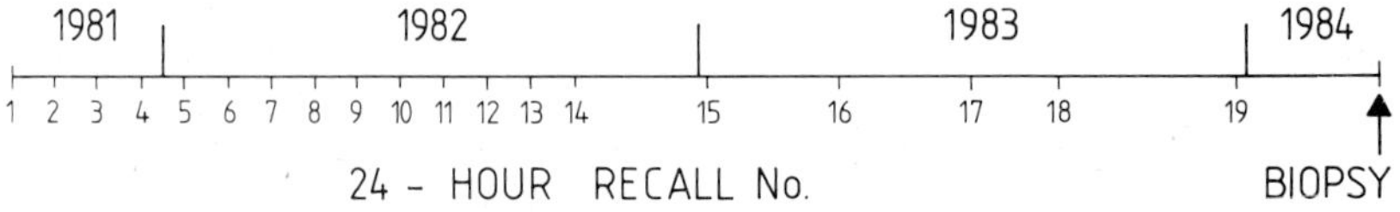

FIGURE 1. Design of the study on linoleic acid in fat tissue biopsies as an indicator of intake (2,5).

over the course of a 2.5 year period using the 24-h recall method. Subsequently, a single microbiopsy of subcutaneous fat was obtained from the buttock in each of them[1]. As shown in Figure 2, there was a strong correlation between the individual values for the intake of linoleic acid and for the proportion in the subcutaneous fat tissue. The intake was assessed as the mean of all 19 recalls performed in each subject. If only a single 24-h recall was used to assess intake – a very common procedure in studies on dietary determinants of disease – then the correlation fell to 0.28. The reason for this difference is well known[3]: a person's intake on a particular day is not at all representative of that person's long-term intake. As a result, many of the intake values obtained by a single recall are grossly in error if the long-term intake is the variable on which information is being sought.

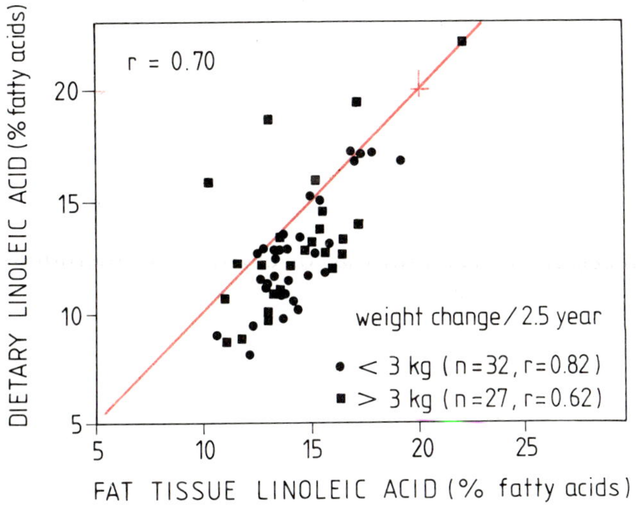

FIGURE 2. Correlation between linoleic acid in the diet, assessed as the mean of 19 recalls per subject (cf Figure 1), and linoleic acid in subcutaneous fat. Separate data are given for those women whose body weight fluctuated by more than 3 kg over the duration of the study (■, and those subjects whose body weight was more stable (●). Reproduced from ref 2, with permission.

Over the past 5 to 10 years, major advances have been made in the technique of capillary gas chromatography. As a result it is now possible to assay the proportion of the highly unsaturated very-long-chain polyunsaturated fatty acid, eicosapentaenoic acid (also known as EPA, timnodonic acid, or C20:5 n-3) in biological samples with great accuracy and reproducibility[4].

Due to the lack of food table data, and the variability of the EPA content in fish, we considered it impossible to obtain reliable estimates of EPA intake by survey in the manner used for linoleic acid above. We have therefore investigated the potential of EPA in blood cells as an indicator of intake by feeding volunteers known amounts of fish oil, and monitoring the rise in EPA in erythrocyte lipids. The amount of EPA supplemented was indeed reflected in the proportion of EPA in the erythrocytes. Equilibrium values were reached between 2 and 6 months after initiation of supplementation. It can be calculated that each increase in erythrocyte EPA by 2 g/100 g fatty acids would reflect an increase in intake by 3.20 0.13 g/d (mean ± SE) over the past 7 days or of 1.24 0.10 g/d over the past few months.

Conclusions

Our data on linoleic acid are in good agreement with those of other workers. They suggest that the adipose tissue content of linoleic acid is a more reliable indicator of a subject's long-term exposure to dietary linoleic acid than the intake as assessed by a single 24-h dietary recall. The data on EPA are encouraging, and suggest new ways to study the relation between exposure to the "fish fatty acids" – and the occurrence of disease. However, more studies are needed before we can be confident that the relation found between EPA intake and erythrocyte EPA levels in the present experiment will also hold for those populations of interest to epidemiologists.

Acknowledgements

We are greatly indebted to our volunteers in Renkum and to the Brothers in Egmond, Oosterhout, Vaals, and Zundert for the selflessness and dedication with which they participated in these studies. In addition we are grateful to Jan Burema MSc, Ans Soffers, Petra van der Wal, Joke Korevaar, and Magda Hectors for their contribution to these investigations, and to the Praeventiefonds, The Hague, The Netherlands and Sanofi-Labaz, Belgium for funding.

References

1 Beynen AC, Katan MB. Rapid sampling and long-term storage of subcutaneous adipose-tissue biopsies for determination of fatty acid composition. Am J Clin Nutr 1985;42:317–22.
2 Beynen AC, Katan MB, Van Staveren WA. The linoleic acid content of subcutaneous adipose tissue as a valid index of the intake of linoleic acid by individuals. Fette Seifen Anstr 1986;88:579–81.
3 Cameron ME, Van Staveren WA, eds. Manual on methodology for food consumption studies. Oxford medical publications, Oxford University Press, 1988.
4 Katan MB, Van de Bovenkamp P. Eicosapentaenoic acid in fat. Lancet 1987;i;862–3.
5 Van Staveren WA, Deurenberg P, Katan MB, Burema J, De Groot CPGM, Hoffmans MDAF. Validity of the fatty acid composition of subcutaneous fat tissue microbiopsies as an estimate of the of the long-term average fatty acid composition of the diet of separate individuals. Am J Epidemiol 1986;123:455–63.

5

Validation of dietary assessment through biomarkers

SHEILA A BINGHAM

MRC and University of Cambridge Dunn Clinical Nutrition Centre, Cambridge, United Kingdom

Introduction

The validity of measurements of dietary intake in free-living individuals is difficult to assess because all methods rely on information given by the subjects themselves, which may not be correct. In an attempt to determine objective measures of validating dietary assessments, the search has begun for objective measures using biological specimens that closely reflect dietary intake, but which do not rely on reports of food consumption[1]. To date, however, there is only a limited number of biomarkers that are sufficiently precise and unbiased in themselves to validate dietary assessments. Two of these are energy expenditure as assessed by the doubly labelled water technique for comparison with energy intake, and the 24 hour urine nitrogen output for comparison with protein intake. These will be discussed, together with shortened approaches.

Doubly-labelled water technique

The doubly-labelled water method is an important advance in the measurement of energy expenditure, since it can be used on free-living individuals with virtually no interference with everyday life, in contrast to previous

Biomarkers of dietary exposure. Ed. F. J. Kok & P. van 't Veer.

procedures. Subjects are given a carefully weighed oral dose of $^{2}H_{2}{}^{18}O$ and are then required only to donate timed urine samples over the next 15 days. Carbon dioxide production is measured as the difference in the water pool (measured by $^{2}H_{2}$) and the bicarbonate plus water pool (measured as ^{18}O). Changes in body weight and the water pool can be used to correct measured energy intake in relation to energy expenditure from the doubly-labelled water method. When this is done, energy expenditure should equal energy intake[15].

In early reports, energy expenditure assessed from this method was unexpectedly low, 1–4 times the basal metabolic rate (BMR) on average in a small group of sedentary women[15]. In normal weight women, energy intake from weighed dietary records agreed with energy expenditure data, but in obese women energy intake assessed from 7 day weighed records was about 2 MJ (465 kcal) lower than expenditure, suggesting that overweight women do not report their habitual food intake[14].

In a more recent study, energy expenditure also exceeded energy intake measured from 7-day records in 31 normal weight individuals, on average by 20%[12]. As a ratio to BMR, energy intake was 1.46 ± 0.31, and energy expenditure 1.82 ± 0.2, greater than previously found in sedentary women[15]. Reports of energy intake were satisfactory, as judged by agreement with energy expenditure, in about a third of these subjects. These were at the higher end of the distribution in energy intake[12].

Schoeller[16] and Black et al. (this symposium) have collated estimates of energy expenditure using the doubly-labelled water method and reports of energy intake from dietary assessments. These show that, in group terms, there is a consistent tendency to under-report food intake. This effect is less obvious in lean subjects, and is not confined to western populations[16]. So far, there is too little information to assess the validity of particular methods of dietary assessment, although Livingstone et al. (this symposium) show that results using the diet history in adolescents were more reliable than those derived from weighed records, at least on a group basis. The high cost of this technique, at least 350 per person for the isotope alone, rules out its use in epidemiology and hence the assessment of individual measures of dietary intake.

24 h urine nitrogen

24 h urine nitrogen is the most well known biological marker, with individual results from published metabolic studies where dietary intake is kept constant over prolonged periods of time showing a fair correlation between daily N intake and daily urine N excretion. Its use depends on the assumption that subjects are in N balance, there being no accumulation due to growth or repair of lost muscle tissue, or loss due to starvation, slimming or injury. This was appreciated as early as 1924, when it was suggested that actual protein intake, as assessed from 24 h urine excretion, was far lower than the recommended level[8].

The apparent accuracy of 24 h urine nitrogen as a biological marker has led to the suggestion that it be used to validate estimates of protein intake from various dietary survey methods[10]. Isaksson[10] summarised a number of studies carried out by his group which showed that estimates of protein intake obtained from 24 h recalls of food intake tended to underestimate when compared with the urine nitrogen, but that estimates from diet histories and food records were in good agreement with the urine values. Van Staveren et al.[19] also found agreement between 24 h urine N and diet history estimates of protein intake. These findings are not consistent however since Van Staveren[19] found little or no under-reporting from the 24 h recall in 123 young females. A recent reanalysis of the Gothenburg work has shown that individuals with a BMI in excess of 24 significantly under-reported their protein intake by the diet history as compared with urine nitrogen[9]. Further studies from this group have confirmed the difficulties of dietary assessments of patients. In obese subjects for example, reported protein intake (from a diet history) was only 46 g but on the basis of 24-hour urine collections it was 87 g[18]. In another study subjects who were overweight or diabetic seemed to report their prescribed diet rather than what they were actually eating as judged by their urine N excretion[22]. Other early comparisons between average urine N and dietary intake have been summarised elsewhere[1]. In general, there is poor agreement between individual estimates of usual protein intake, and the 24 h urine N output.

The reasons for this poor agreement are three-fold, in addition to inaccuracies in dietary assessment. First, it is clearly inappropriate to attempt to "validate" estimates of diet with urine collections unless these collections are shown to be complete, or to replace dietary estimates with a less accurate biological marker. Total 24 h urine creatinine is sometimes used as a measure of completeness of 24 h urine collections, and its output is probably constant when individuals are fed constant diets[21]. However, urinary creatinine is not constant when a normal ad lib diet is consumed because of the creatinine content of cooked meat[11]. The pool size of creatinine is small, hence ingested creatinine is quickly excreted, leading to a 70% range in 24 h excretion, even after taking variations in fat free mass into account[2]. Daily variability in fact is not significantly less than that in total N or urea[6], and there therefore seems little justification for attempting to use creatinine for the purposes of validating dietary estimates.

Because of these problems, the PABA (para-amino-benzoic acid) marker was developed as a check on the completeness of 24 h urine collections[2]. The method consists of 3 tablets of 80 mg PABA taken with meals that are quantitatively excreted within 24 hours, so that single collections containing less than 85% of the PABA marker can be classified as unsatisfactory, either because the tablets have not been taken, or because one or more specimens was omitted from the collection.

Further sources of error are the extent of extrarenal losses of nitrogen, and lack of precision from too few observations of either dietary intake or urine excretion. These were investigated in a study of 8 individuals eating their normal diet, but whilst they were making faecal and urine collections validated for their completeness with radio-opaque markers and PABA over a 28 day period. Duplicates of all food eaten were taken for nitrogen analysis, and skin and blood losses measured[3]. Extrarenal losses varied from individual to individual and were greater at higher levels of protein intake than lower ones. Hence the urine nitrogen underestimates at high levels of protein intake and overestimates at lower levels if a constant factor for faecal and skin losses is used. This can be overcome by expressing the urine values as a proportion of dietary intake, which on average is 80%. The limits of precision of this value depend on numbers of observations on each individual, or the numbers of individuals in the group for single collections. The extent of daily variation is such that individuals are rarely in nitrogen balance so that on a day to day, basis, urine nitrogen is poorly correlated with N intake. The expected correlations between daily intake and output are in the region of 0.5 when single days data are used, with a low estimate of precision, coefficient of variation 24%. When 8 days urine collections and 18 days dietary observations are available, the correlation improves to 0.95, and the coefficient of variation to 5%. Several 24 h collections, validated fore their completeness are therefore required to make accurate comparisons with dietary intake data, the exact number depending on the precision required. With an average coefficient of variation of 13% in urine N excretion, 8 days of collections will estimate N output to within ±5% standard error[3].

In an ongoing study of the validity of various methods of dietary assessment in individuals in Cambridge, subjects are asked to weigh their food using PETRA scales for four days and to collect 24 h urine samples once weighing their food and once when not weighing their food. The completeness of the urine samples is assessed by the PABAcheck method. Subjects are asked to repeat this four times per year and so far 80 subjects have been studied. Body weight is also obtained, together with a fasting blood and breath sample, at each dietary season.

The importance of including a measure of the completeness of the urine collections themselves is shown in Table 1, where data from another epidemiological study[23] and some clinical work[4] has been collated with that from the above study. In urines which have been classified as incomplete, there are systematically lower contents of nearly all analytes compared with those that are complete. The consistently lower values for nitrogen are particularly important from the point of dietary validation, since it shows that omission of an objective check on 24 h urine collections in a dietary validation study will underestimate the extent of bias in a dietary assessment method.

On completion of the study, the average N intake from the 16 days of records has been compared with the average N excretion in the complete 24 h urine collections, with the expected ratio of urine N to dietary N being 81 ± 5%[3]. 34 of the 79 individuals excreted more than two standard deviations in excess of the expected ratio of 81% (91%) of their reported dietary N intake in urine, and were classified as 'under-reporters'. Of these 8 lost from

TABLE 1. Analytes in complete versus incomplete 24h urine collections.

		Mean	Standard deviation	Significance of difference
Specimens collected by hospital outpatients				
Volume	1[a]	1788	663	
(ml)	2	1692	971	ns
PABA	1	94	6	
(%)	2	70	12	
Potassium	1	63	19	
(mmol)	2	56	13	ns
Sodium	1	134	51	
(mmol)	2	103	51	0.03
Creatinine	1	10.8	3.0	
(mmol)	2	9.3	2.7	0.06
Urea	1	301	78	
(mmol)	2	223	63	0.001
Nitrogen	1	10.1	2.7	
(g)	2	8.3	2.4	0.01
Specimens collected by randomly selected healthy men				
PABA	1[b]	95	6	
(%)	2	69	9	
Potassium	1	74	23	
(mmol)	2	66	15	ns
Sodium	1	172	52	
(mmol)	2	131	31	0.001
Urea	1	380	104	
(mmol)	2	281	64	0.001
Specimens collected by 50–60 y women				
PABA	1[c]	97	7	
(%)	2	69	15	
Potassium	1	72	22	
(mmol)	2	61	20	0.001
Sodium	1	109	36	
(mmol)	2	111	36	ns
Nitrogen	1	10.4	2.7	
(g)	2	9.2	2.4	0.001

1[a] 'Complete' group: 30 female, 15 male patients, total 45 collections, duration 23.6 ± 0.6 h.
2 'Incomplete' group: 9 female, 9 male patients, total 18 collections, duration 23.5 ± 1.0 h.
1[b] 'Complete' group: 71 men, duration 23.5 ± 2.2 h.
2 'Incomplete' group: 12 men, duration 21.7 ± 5.0 h.
1[c] 'Complete' group: 445 women, nitrogen;
308 women, sodium and potassium
2 'Incomplete' group: 208 women, nitrogen;
185 women, sodium and potassium

TABLE 2. Differences between under-reporters and other subjects mean and (sd)

Numbers	Under-reporters 34		Others 45		p<
Urine N/diet N[a]	1.07	(0.15)	0.81	(0.07)	
Weight kg	75	(13)	62	(8)	.001
Height m	1.66	(0.06)	1.63	(0.07)	.05
W/H^2 kg/m^2	26.8	(4.5)	23.3	(3.0)	.01
EI/BMRb	1.21	(0.24)	1.58	(0.21)	.0001
Energy MJ	7.01	(1.22)	8.70	(1.24)	.0001
Protein g	65	(11)	73	(11)	.003
Fat g	65	(15)	87	(14)	.0001
Fat % energy	35.3	(4.7)	38.1	(4.3)	.001
Tot sugars g	92	(29)	127	(32)	.0001
Added sugars g	37	(22)	58	(28)	.0001
Starch g	103	(25)	113	(24)	ns
NSP (dietary fibre) g	14	(6)	15	(5)	ns
Alcohol g	8	(10)	9	(16)	ns
Vitamin C mg	91	(33)	103	(36)	ns

[a]Ratio of urine nitrogen (g) from complete 24 h specimens to daily intake of nitrogen (g) from 16 days weighed records;
[b]Ratio energy intake in MJ to basal metabolic rate calculated from equations in Table 3.

2–4 kg body weight over the year, but 7 gained 2–4 kg. No changes occurred in the other 19 subjects[5].

Table 2 compares daily dietary intake data and body weight (mean and standard deviation) for the 34 under-reporters and 45 other subjects. The 'under-reporters' were significantly heavier than the other subjects and differences were evident between average reported intakes of energy, protein, fat and sugars from records obtained from under-reporters and those subjects whose records appeared to be valid from the 24 h urine nitrogen. There were no differences in alcohol, NSP and starch consumption.

Hence, bias in reports of food intake obtained from weighed dietary records can be detected by the use of 24 h urine nitrogen. Simultaneous use of both the 24 h urine N and doubly-labelled water has shown that both methods identify the same subjects who under-report their food intake when asked to keep weighed records (Fig. 1; 7). Only some, not all, nutrients may be under-reported and the range of individual values within the distribution will be artefactually extended. Figure 2, for example, shows the distribution of reported intakes of fat where it can be seen that under-recording has a particular effect on the distribution of the absolute intake of fat, although there is less truncation of the distribution when expressed as a proportion of total energy.

In this survey, under-reporting was more likely to occur in overweight individuals, and could have arisen either from failure to report all food eaten during the 16-day period, or because the subjects decided to diet

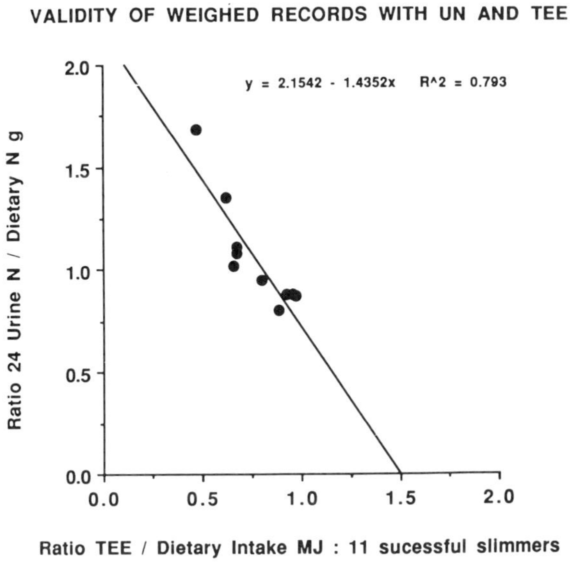

FIGURE 1. Ratio total energy expenditure (from doubly-labelled water technique) to dietary intake (from weighed records) MJ to ratio 24 hour urine N (from complete 24h urine specimens) to dietary N intake (from weighed records) g in 11 successful slimmers (From Black et al.: ref 7)

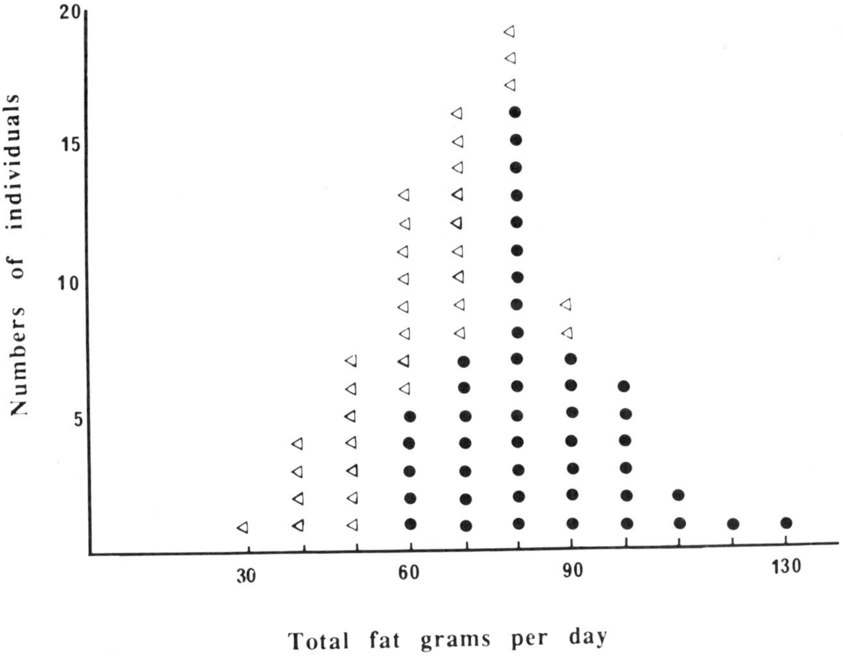

FIGURE 2. Distribution of total daily dietary fat (g) in 86 volunteer women aged 50–65 measured over 16 days by weighed food records using the PETRA system.
Open symbols = "under-reporters" as judged by 24h urine nitrogen excretion.

whilst weighing their food, causing a negative nitrogen balance. Adiposity may not be a universal predictor of the tendency to under-report, Livingstone et al.[12] finding no association between body mass index and the extent of under-reporting from the 7-day weighed record assessed by the doubly-labelled water method.

Body weight

A simple check on the validity of group estimates is to weigh subjects, and to calculate basal metabolic rate from the equations shown in Table 3[17]. Table 3 also shows the WHO allowances for sedentary and more active lifestyles, but in most western populations an allowance of 1.6 times BMR is more than adequate for total energy expenditure. Table 2 shows that this was the value obtained in subjects who gave valid estimates of their dietary intakes from weighed records, as judged by the 24 h urine nitrogen test. Another simple test is to weigh subjects before and after periods of record keeping. Over a 4-day period of weighed intake for example, a systematic loss of 0.3 ± 0.7 kg ($p < 0.01$) in 80 women occurred, despite the fact that the weights were not obtained under standard conditions (Bingham et al. unpublished).

TABLE 3a. Equations for estimated basal metabolic rate from weight (m male, f female). (BMR is expressed in MJ/24h; weight in kg; sample size is given as n; multiple correlation as R; standard error of the estimate as s.e.).

Children: under 3 years	n	R	s.e.
m BMR = 0.249 wt - 0.127	162	0.95	0.2925
f BMR = 0.244 wt - 0.130	137	0.96	0.2456
3 to 10 years			
m BMR = 0.095 wt + 2.110	338	0.83	0.2803
f BMR = 0.085 wt + 2.033	413	0.81	0.2924
10 to 18 years			
m BMR = 0.074 wt + 2.754	734	0.93	0.4404
f BMR = 0.056 wt + 2.898	575	0.80	0.4661
Adults: 18 to 30 years			
m BMR = 0.063 wt + 2.896	2879	0.65	0.6407
f BMR = 0.062 wt + 2.036	829	0.73	0.4967
30 to 60 years			
m BMR = 0.048 wt + 3.653	646	0.60	0.6997
f BMR = 0.034 wt + 3.538	372	0.68	0.4653
Over 60 years			
m BMR = 0.049 wt + 2.459	50	0.71	0.6865
f BMR = 0.038 wt + 2.755	38	0.68	0.4511

(From Schofield et al.: ref 17)

TABLE 3b. Average daily energy requirements of adults whose occupational work is classified as light, moderate, or heavy expressed as a multiple of BMR

	Light	Moderate	Heavy
Men	1.55	1.78	2.10
Women	1.56	1.64	1.82

(From WHO: ref 24)

Neither of these tests is sufficiently precise for individual validations, due to normal fluctuations in body weight, to individual variations in BMR calculated from body weight (coefficient of variation ± 12%), and variations in activity levels. Energy intakes less than 1.2 × the calculated BMR can probably be excluded from analyses with certainty as erroneous estimates of habitual food intake. Greater accuracy in predicting cut-off values is not however possible in the absence of accurate measures of BMR and energy expenditure.

Urea and potassium

Urine urea is a constant proportion (85%) of total nitrogen excretion when individuals are consuming normal mixed western diets and are in overall nitrogen balance[3]. It could therefore replace the estimation of total N in these circumstances and is considerably easier to analyse. As a proportion of total N intake, 24 h urine urea N is 70 ± 7%, and urea plus creatinine N 73 ± 7% of the habitual diet when eight 24 h collections are obtained. Problems would be encountered at lower levels of protein consumption, when urea would be a smaller proportion of total N output.

Table 4 shows calculated average intakes from 8 subjects and urines excretion of nitrogen, urea, potassium and sodium, obtained from 24 h urines validated for their completeness with the PABA technique, averaged over a 28-day period[3]. Extra renal losses of potassium are similar to those of nitrogen, and the correlations between dietary intake and excretion are of the same order. However, the within person variation is approximately two times greater for potassium excretion than it is for nitrogen or urea, so that greater numbers of collections from each individual would be required. Potassium is widely distributed in foods, but the lack of precision from 24 h urine output limits its use as a biological marker for validation purposes. As such it has not been used for the purposes of assessing the accuracy of dietary survey techniques in individuals.

Despite the high correlation between urine sodium and calculated dietary intake (Table 4), the regression coefficient deviates appreciably from unity. 24 h urine is routinely used to assess sodium consumption, but it is clearly inappropriate for validation purposes due to interference with discretionary use of salt.

TABLE 4. Urinary validation markers[a].

	Urine N g	Urea N g	K mmol	Na mmol
Average urine	12.9	10.9	89	128
Average diet	16.0	16.0	112	138
Ratio %	81	68	79	93
Intra Urine cv%[b]	14	15	24	30
Inter Urine cv%[b]	24	25	21	12
Ratio	0.6	0.6	1.2	2.5
Slope	1.36	1.61	1.21	1.61
Correlation coefficient diet v. urine values	0.99	0.99	0.96	0.95

[a] (From Bingham and Cummings: ref 3)
[b] (From Bingham et al.: ref 6)

Partial urine collections

Due to the difficulty of obtaining complete 24 h collections, and the lack of precision of single ones, replacement with partial collections has been investigated. Yamori et al.[25] obtained 24 h collections split into four time periods from 16 volunteer medical students and the variation of urea and creatinine in relation to the full 24 h period are shown in Table 5, together with the correlation coefficients between separate samples and 24 h ones. Values for overnight collections in relation to full 24 h collections obtained from 21 men and women aged 19 to 65 y from the study of Ogawa[13] are also shown.

TABLE 5. Partial collections in relation to 24 h urine collections.

Time of urine collection	Daily variation in 24 h[a]		Correlation with 24		
	Urea N	Urea/Creatinine ratio	Urea N	Urea/Creatinine ratio	
Morning	101 (34)	103 (33)	0.63	0.72	
Afternoon	122 (36)	111 (39)	0.72	0.50	
Evening	114 (44)	106 (44)	0.78	0.81	
Overnight	74 (27)	86 (29)	0.76	0.81	0.77[b]
24 h	100 (26)	100 (23)			

[a] Mean (sd) of all samples, converted so that the mean values in the 24 h samples equals 100 (From Yamori et al.: ref 25)
[b] (From Ogawa et al.: ref 13)

From this, it would seem that overnight collections contain both less urea and a lower urea to creatinine ratio than others, whereas afternoon values are higher. Correlation coefficients are of the same order for both evening and overnight collections. It is possible that the proportion of constituents in partial collections varies, as indicated by the relatively large standard deviations in Table 2, probably depending on the timing of diet and main meal consumption. This is probably true also of different populations, so that it is not possible to make general statements of the utility of partial collections, other than they are far less accurate than full 24 h collections for estimating protein intake. The possibility of increasing accuracy by repeat partial collections requires investigation in sub-samples of the population of interest.

Conclusions

The doubly-labelled water and 24 h urine nitrogen technique are well investigated biological markers that are sufficiently accurate to use as validatory measures in dietary surveys. The limited information available so far suggests that they are probably closely related and interchangeable, in that both can document under-reporting of usual food intake in free-living individuals. However, under-reporting by a proportion of individuals leads to bias in the overall average for some, but not all, nutrients. Available evidence suggests that fat and sucrose are under-reported, but not micronutrients such as vitamin C for example.

Under-reporting by a proportion of individuals artefactually extends the range of nutrient values within a group. This has profound implications for analytic studies in nutritional epidemiology. The limited data available suggests that all methods of dietary assessment are prone to this problem, and that it is not confined to any particular method such as records of food consumption.

Estimated energy intake from body weight can be used to demonstrate bias in a group assessment of energy intake, but there are limitations as to the value of this, and other shortened methods, for individuals.

References

1 Bingham SA. The dietary assessment of individuals: methods, accuracy, new techniques and recommendations. Nutr Abs & Rev 1987;57:705–742.

2 Bingham SA, Cummings JH. The use of 4-amino benzoic acid as a marker to validate the completeness of 24h urine collections in man. Clin Sci 1983;64:629–635.

3 Bingham SA, Cummings JH. Urine nitrogen as an independent validatory measure of dietary intake. Am J Clin Nutr 1985;42:1276–1289.

4 Bingham SA, Murphy J, Waller L, Runswick S, et al. Incomplete 24h urine collections from hospital out-patients. Submitted for publication. 1991.

5 Bingham SA, Welch A, Cassidy A, Runswick S, et al. 24h urine used to detect bias in reported food intake of individuals assessed from weighed dietary records (Abstract). Proc Nutr Soc 1991 (in press).

6 Bingham SA, Williams R, Cole TJ, Price CP, Cummings JH. Reference values for analytes of 24-h urine collections known to be complete. Ann Clin Biochem 1988;25:610–619.

7 Black A, Parkinson S, Bingham SA. Validation of energy and protein intakes assessed by diet history and by weighed diet records against total energy expenditure and 24h urine nitrogen (Abstract). Proc Nutr Soc 1991 (in press).
8 Denis W, Borgstrom P. A study of the effect of temperature on protein intake. J Biol Chem 1924;61:109–116.
9 Hulten B, Bengtsson C, Isaksson B. Some errors inherent in a longitudinal dietary survey. Eur J Clin Nutr 1990;44:169–174.
10 Isaksson B. Urinary nitrogen output as a validity test in dietary surveys. Am J Clin Nutr 1980;33:4–6.
11 Jacobsen FK, Christensen CK, Morgensen CE, Andreason F, Heilskov NS. Pronounced increase in serum cholesterol after eating cooked meat. Br Med J 1979;i:1049–1050.
12 Livingstone MBE, Prentice AM, Strain JJ, Coward WA, et al. Accuracy of weighed dietary records in studies of diet and health. Br Med J 1990;300:708–712.
13 Ogawa M. Feasibility of overnight urine for assessing dietary intakes of sodium, potassium, protein and sulphur amino acids in field studies. Jap Circ J 1986;50:595–600.
14 Prentice AM, Black AE, Coward WA, Davies HL, et al. High levels of energy expenditure in obese women. Br Med J 1986;292:983–987.
15 Prentice AM, Coward WA, Davies HL, Murgatroyd PR, et al. Unexpectedly low levels of energy expenditure in healthy women. Lancet 1985;ii:1419–1422.
16 Schoeller DA How accurate is self-reported dietary energy intake? Nutr Rev 1990;49:373–379.
17 Schofield WN, Schofield C, James WPT. Basal metabolic rate. Human Nutr: Clin Nutr 1985;39C,Suppl.1:1–96.
18 Steen B, Isaksson B, Svanborg A. Intake of energy and nutrients and meal habits in 70 year old males and females in Gothenburg, Sweden: a population study. Acta Med Scand 1977;Suppl.611:39–86.
19 Van Staveren WA. Food intake measurements: their validity and reproducibility. PhD Thesis, Wageningen University. 1985.
20 Van Staveren WA, de Boer JO, Burema J. Validity and reproducibility of a diet history method estimating the usual food intake during one month. Am J Clin Nutr 1985;42:554–559.
21 Vestergaard P, Leverett MS, Orangeburg NY. Constancy of urinary creatinine excretion. J Lab Clin Med 1958;51:211–218.
22 Warnold I, Carlgren G, Krotkiewski M. Energy expenditure and body composition during weight reduction in hyperplastic obese women. Am J Clin Nutr 1978;31:750–763.
23 Williams DRR, Bingham SA. Sodium and potassium intakes in a representative population sample: estimates from 24h urine collections known to be complete. Br J Nutr 1986;55:13–22.
24 World Health Organisation Energy and protein requirements. Tech. Rep. Ser. 724, WHO, Geneva. 1985.
25 Yamori Y, Kihara M, Fujikawa J, et al. Dietary risk factors for stroke in Japan. Jap Circ J 1982;46: 933–938.

6

Biomarkers of mutagenic and carcinogenic dietary exposure

DAVID FORMAN

Cancer Epidemiology Unit, University of Oxford, Imperial Cancer Research Fund, Oxford, United Kingdom

Introduction

Most of the biomarkers considered at this meeting are being used as indicators of external exposure to (or intake of) dietary nutrients. Such biomarkers will, of course, also be of value for future research into the aetiology of cancer. It is also possible to exploit other categories of biomarkers that can be indicative of "internal dose" or "biologically effective exposures". Such biomarkers (or molecular dosimeters) may be thought of, to varying degrees, as integrating external exposures with such factors as host defence mechanisms, metabolic activation systems and concurrent exposures to catalytic or inhibitory agents. The hope is that these biomarkers may be more biologically relevant than markers of exposure *per se*. It is perhaps understandable that cancer research should be an area in which advances in these methods have been made, given the rapid developments in our understanding of cellular and biochemical changes that preceed tumour development. Most of the best examples of such approaches in cancer "molecular epidemiology" are, however, from occupational studies and there are relatively few pertinent examples in dietary research.

The four examples that follow represent a variety of technical procedures that have been employed in assaying biomarkers of mutagenic and carcino-

Biomarkers of dietary exposure. Ed. F. J. Kok & P. van 't Veer.

genic dietary exposures eg. Enzyme Linked Immuno Sorbent Assay (ELISA) systems, competitive enzyme repair, Gas Chromatography (GC)-thermal energy analysis and direct visualisation of nuclear damage. They also represent different methodological approaches that can be used. These can be highly specific eg. direct measurement of individual mutagens or carcinogens or more general eg. use of "surrogate" biomarkers to represent exposure to a general class of mutagens or carcinogens, or biomarkers that indicate DNA damaging effects.

Exposure to aflatoxins

The first example is of a biomarker to indicate the level of exposure to aflatoxins. The aflatoxins are a group of metabolites of the fungus *Aspergillus Flavus,* a widespread contaminant of cereal crops in developing countries. The aflatoxins have potent hepatotoxic and hepatocarcinogenic effects and have been classified by the International Agency for Research on Cancer as Class I carcinogens (ie. with sufficient evidence of human carcinogenicity). In the past, estimates of individual intake have been notoriously unreliable and have relied largely on assessing cereal intake and measuring aflatoxin levels in the crops. It has therefore been impossible to individually monitor "at risk" populations or to examine dose-response characteristics of exposure. Also, until recently, the epidemiological evidence underlying the assessment of aflatoxin as a human carcinogen has depended on ecological studies in which cereal crop contamination has been compared in different geographical regions with contrasting liver cancer mortality rates. Although this evidence has been highly consistent it conflicts with more recent studies in which exposure has been assessed by measuring aflatoxin adducts in individual urine samples[2]. This has opened up a debate about how reliable the evidence is concerning the carcinogenicity of aflatoxin. It is not the purpose here to weigh up this evidence but to make the point that the reason for the uncertainty is due to a lack of reliable human exposure data. There is available now a method for the detection of the aflatoxin B1 adduct bound to serum or plasma albumin[7] which should help improve the situation. This method, which is ELISA based, is extremely sensitive, highly specific and requires a fingerprick blood sample. It is known that albumin binding parallels binding to hepatocyte DNA and albumin adducts indicate exposure over a period of weeks or months (unlike urinary adducts that indicate exposure over days). Although yet to be used in extensive epidemiological studies the albumin assay offers the prospect of resolving unanswered questions about aflatoxin carcinogenicity.

Test for *N*-nitroso compounds

The second example is the *N*-nitrosoproline (NPRO) test originally devised by Ohshima and Bartsch[5] ten years ago. The NPRO test measures urinary NPRO in a 12 or 24 hour urine sample after ingestion of a loading dose of proline. In theory, the test indicates an individual's propensity for undergoing endogenous nitrosation, ie. the formation of endogenous *N*-nitroso compounds after ingestion of dietary precursors. Many *N*-nitroso compounds are highly carcinogenic and it has been suggested that exposure to them is an important risk factor for oesophageal and gastric cancers. A major problem has been determining the level of exposure to such endogenously synthesised compounds. Assessment of precursors, such as dietary nitrate or secondary amines, has always been thought to be inadequate as so many other factors (exogenous eg. vitamin C, smoking and endogenous eg. gastric pH) are known to affect synthesis. Assessment of the resulting *N*-nitroso compounds themselves has been technically extremely difficult and the results unreliable. The NPRO-test was an ingenious attempt to overcome these problems by measuring the extent to which exogenous proline is nitrosated to form NPRO. This is excreted unmetabolised in urine and can be reliably estimated with high sensitivity using GC-Thermal Energy Analysis. NPRO itself is neither carcinogenic or mutagenic (and thus the test is ethically acceptable) but its formation may act as a general marker of nitrosation potential. It has now been used in epidemiological studies to test whether specific cancers are associated with nitrosation (1) and also to examine which dietary factors effect NPRO formation. Again the purpose here is not to review this research but to demonstrate one solution to a complex problem of dietary exposure.

Detection of alkyl-DNA adducts

The third example is the detection of alkyl-DNA adducts in lymphocytes. Certain of these adducts, eg 0^6-me-guanine, are mutagenic and DNA with a methyl (or other alkyl) group at the 0^6 site of guanine is believed to be an important precarcinogenic lesion. Alkylating agents which can cause this adduct to be formed are often of dietary origin and thus detection of these adducts offers a "global" indicator of exposure to such agents. Animal studies have shown that alkylating agents which can cause cancer in specific organs produce adducts in both the target organ and in peripheral blood lymphocyte DNA and that there is a quantitative relationship between the extent of adduct formation at both sites. Thus it is possible to use lymphocyte DNA as a general monitor of exposure. There is also a quantitative proportionality between mutagenic adducts and other non-mutagenic adducts, eg. N^7-me-guanine, which are formed in greater abundance and are thus easier to assess. Assessment of alkylated DNA can make direct use of molecular techniques which enables extremely high levels of sensitivity. Thus an assay for 0^6-me-guanine based on competitive enzymatic DNA repair can detect as little as 50 femtomoles 0^6-me-guanine per mg DNA using 10–15 micrograms of DNA[6]. This topic will be dealt with in greater detail in the paper by Hemminki.

Scoring of micronuclei

The fourth and final example is more of a model biomarker system for human experimental studies than an epidemiological tool. It involves the detection of micronucleated erythrocytes in peripheral blood[3]. This provides an index of chromosomal damage in erythrocyte precursor cells which is, in turn, related to cancer risk. Nucleated erythrocytes can only be detected in humans who have had a splenectomy and this is an obvious major constraint in their use. Nevertheless in such individuals, usually traffic accident survivors, erythrocytes can be used to investigate rapidly the clastogenic effects of diet and other factors. Fingerprick blood samples can be used and the visual scoring of micronuclei is relatively simple and can be automated. Also one can distinguish between immature and fully mature erythrocytes in which the presence of micronuclei indicates exposures to damaging agents over periods of days and months respectively. A similar assay can be carried out in lymphocytes but it is much less sensitive than the erythrocyte assay and require larger blood samples. Preliminary studies show a strong effect of folate deficiency on micronuclei formation which is reversible by folate supplementation[3]. Also vitamin supplementation appears to reduce significantly the extent of micronuclei formation[4].

Conclusions

These examples, in different ways, show the advantages and problems of using molecular biomarkers in nutritional epidemiology. They can certainly provide biologically relevant exposure with a high level of sensitivity. At the same time there can be practical and methodological constraints to their utility. Such markers are, therefore, powerful tools but they are not instant solutions and they require application in well-designed epidemiological studies. In particular, it should be emphasised that problem of confounding, bias and multiple hypothesis testing are as relevant to biomarker epidemiology as they are to questionnaire-based studies.

At a more general level, many of these markers reflect short-term transient exposures and have tended to be used in relatively weak ecological study designs. Therefore it does not automatically follow that epidemiological studies are more precise as a result of employing such biomarkers. It still remains essential to interpret results in a correct manner and to acknowledge the limitations of the methodology used in the study.

References

1 Bartsch H, Ohshima H, Pignatelly B, Calmelf F. Human exposure to endogenous *N*-nitroso compounds. Quantitative estimates in subjects at high risk for cancer of the oral cavity, oesophagus, stomac and urinary bladder. Cancer Surv 1989;8:335–362.

2 Campbell TC, Chen J, Liu C, Li J, Parpia B. Nonassociation of aflatoxin with primary liver cancer in a cross-sectional ecological survey in the people's republic of China. Cancer Res 1990;50:6882–93.

3 Everson RB, Wehr CM, Erexson GL, MacGregor JT. Association of marginal folate depletion with increased human chromosomal damage in vivo: demonstration by analysis of micronucleated erythrocytes. J Natl Cancer Inst 1988;80:525–29.

4 MacGregor JT. Dietary factors affecting spontanous chromosomal damage in man. In: Mutagens and carcinogens in the diet. Pariza MW et al. (eds). New York: Wiley 1990:139–153.

5 Ohshima H, Bartsch H. Quantitative estimation of endogenous nitrosation in humans by monitoring *N*-nitrosoproline excreted in the urine. Cancer Res 1981;41:3658–62.
6 Souliotis VL, Kyrtopoulos SA. A novel, sensitive assay for 0^6-methyl-and 0^6-ethylguanine in DNA, based on repair by the enzyme 0^6-alkylguanine-DNA-alkyltransferase in competition with an oligonucleotide containing 0^6-methylguanine. Cancer Res 1989;49:6997–7001.
7 Wild CP, Jiang Y, Sabbioni G, Chapot B, Montesano R. Evaluation of methods for quantitation of aflatoxin-albumin adducts and their application to human exposure assessment. Cancer Res 1990;50:245–51.

7

Application of DNA adduct measurements for dietary studies

KARI HEMMINKI[1,2], R MUSTONEN[1], A REUNANEN[1] and H KAHN[3]

[1]Institute of Occupational Health, Helsinki, Finland
[2]Centre for Nutrition and Toxicology, Huddinge, Sweden
[3]Estonian Center of Occupational Health, Estonia, USSR

Introduction

Diet is assumed to be related to a large proportion of cancer[3,13]. Diet may be involved through a number of mechanisms and affect a number of stages in the multistage transformation of normal cells to tumor cells. It may contain carcinogenic chemicals such as mycotoxins, N-nitrosocompounds, polycyclic aromatic hydrocarbons (PAHs) and heterocyclic amines, which directly react with DNA. As a second mechanism, diet may contain precursors, such as secondary amines and nitrite, which can lead to a formation of carcinogens, in this case nitrosamines, in the body. As a third mechanism, diet may contain chemicals that induce metabolic reactions leading to endogenous formation of DNA-reactive intermediates. Lipid peroxidation is one such process, thought to lead to formation of reactive aldehydes such as malonaldehyde and 4-hydroxy-2-nonenal, both capable of binding to DNA. As a forth mechanism diet may be deficient in factors involved in the inactivation of carcinogenic intermediates in the body, antioxidants, vitamins and microelements. These are mechanisms, which may affect damage to DNA, but undoubtedly other types of mechanisms, e.g., those affecting cell growth rate, are involved.

Biomarkers of dietary exposure. Ed. F. J. Kok & P. van 't Veer.

In the present article we show examples of the application of the ^{32}P-postlabeling technique[7,20–22] to the study of adducts in humans. So far no specific diet-related DNA-adduct has been demonstrated in humans but there are reasons to believe that at least some of the adducts found in all humans are either diet-derived or formed endogenously.

Model compounds for postlabeling

One of the problems of the P-postlabeling technique is that the adduct spots are not readily identifiable. However, by preparing standard compounds and by demonstrating cochromatography chemical identification may be possible.

We have synthesized and obtained from colleagues a number of adduct standards for postlabeling. Most of them are derivatives of 2'-deoxyguanosine 3'-monophosphate (dGMP), which are phosphorylated in the postlabeling reaction by T4 polynucleotide kinase to the corresponding 2'-deoxyguanosine 3'-, 5'-bisphosphates.

We have synthesized N-7-methyl-dGMP and its bisphosphate analog, and shown that the product of postlabeling of N-7-methyl-dGMP in fact cochromatographs with the bisphosphate standard[8]. It is also important to ensure the completeness of the postlabeling reaction, i.e. phosphorylation of all the substrate. In the case of N-7-methyl-dGMP the labeling efficiency is close to 100%, which will make it a good marker adduct in human studies[8].

A group of possibly diet-related standard compounds, N1-N^2-cyclic dGMP derivative of 4-hydroxy-2-nonanal and 2,3-epoxy-4-hydroxynonanal were obtained from Drs RS Sodum and F-L Chung[24,25]. Compound I (Figure 1) is etheno-dGMP and compounds II-VI dGMP substitution products of 2,3-epoxy-4-hydroxynonanal, all possible lipid-peroxidation products. We have studied their labeling efficiency (Figure 1), which is generally high. Compounds I, II and IV are labeled to about 100% in fmol amounts[9]. These would provide good markers for studies on DNA-adduct formation by lipid peroxidation.

N-7-methyl dGMP in humans

Methylation of the N-7 position of guanine in DNA can be caused by a number of agents such as methylating nitrosamines and S-adenosylmethionine. Methylating agents procarbazine and dacarbazine are used in the chemotherapy of cancer. We have studied cancer patients and healthy nonsmoking individuals, and measured the levels of their N-7-methyl-dGMP levels in white blood cell DNA.

The main technical difficulty was to isolate N-7-methyl-dGMP from unmodified nucleotides in order to ensure efficient postlabeling. This was achieved by anion exchange chromatography prior to postlabeling[14]. Figure 2 shows the two-dimensional autoradiograms of DNA from a cancer patient (A) and a healthy individual (B). The phosphorylated N-7-methyl-dGMP was clearly visible in

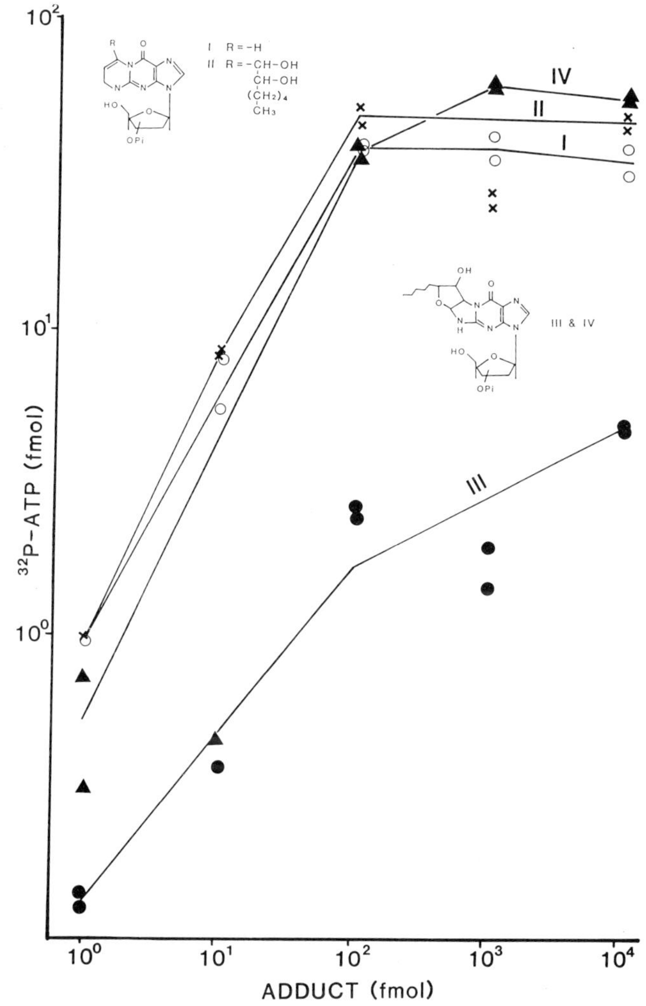

FIGURE 1. Concentration dependence of phosphorylation of cyclic N, N-dGMP adducts, I = etheno-dGMP, II, III and IV dGMP substitution products of 2,3-epoxy-4-hydroxynonanal (or 4-hydroxy-2-nonenal, refs 24,25). The abscissa is the amount of the standard compound added and the ordinate the amount of radioactive product recovered (ref 9).

the patient DNA but not in normal DNA, at the exposure time used. Table 1 summarized the results after quantitation of the appropriate adducts by Cerenkov counting. The mean level of N-7-methyl-dGMP adducts in the patients was 57 per 10^7 normal nucleotides; in healthy individuals the adduct levels were 2.4 per 10^7 normal nucleotides. The total dose regimen in the patients varied between 1050 and 2800 mg, which were delivered in daily doses of 150-200 mg. The adduct levels in the patient varied about 3-fold. The background levels in the healthy individuals varied about 10 times.

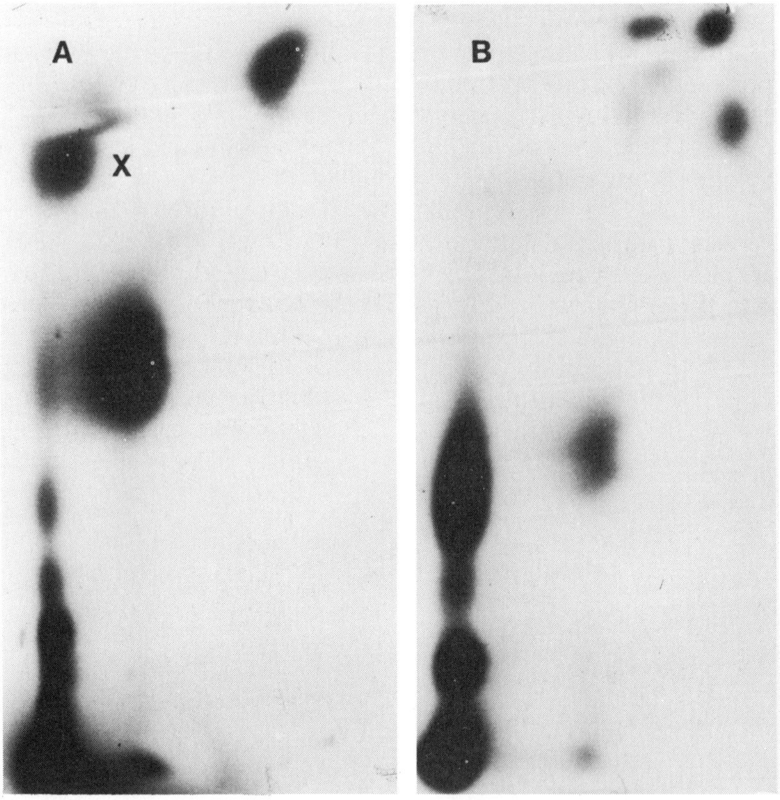

FIGURE 2. Two-dimensional thin-layer-chromatography (TLC) of purified N-7-methyl-dGMP (marked as "X" from white blood cells of a cancer patient (A) and healthy control person (B) after ^{32}P-postlabelings with T4 polynucleotide kinase. TLC was developed with 1 M ammonium formate, pH 5.3 (dimension 1) and 0.5 M LiCl (dimension 2). The radioactive spots were visualized by autoradiography.

TABLE 1. N-7-methyl-dGMP levels in patients treated with procarbazine and dacarbazine, and in healthy individuals (ref. 15).

Group	N	N-7-methyl-dGMP per 10^7 nucleotides
Patients	4	57
Healthy individuals	17	2.4

Aromatic adducts in humans

A study was undertaken in Estonia with an aim to study the possible environmental health problems around the shale oil industry in eastern Estonia[10]. Aromatic adducts of white blood cell DNA were analysed in three populations: shale oil workers, residents in a polluted village, Saka, near the shale oil industry and controls from Tallinn, not known to have occupational exposures to carcinogenic compounds. The results gave some evidence on elevated adducts levels in one sample of the Sake villagers, as will be reported elsewhere. However, interesting features were seen in the autoradiograms from the villagers, possibly related to pollution. It should be pointed out that exposure to polyaromatic compounds is mainly through food due to environmental contamination, holding true even for smokers[28].

Two samples were obtained from the same individuals living in the village close to the polluting industries. The first sampling was in November, that happened to be one of the coldest times of the whole winter. The second sampling was in December, a year later. In the first sampling there were typical spots in autoradiograms, marked as "c" in Figure 3A. These typical spots had disappeared in the second samples taken 12.5 months later, and new spots marked as "d" and "e" emerged (Figure 3B).

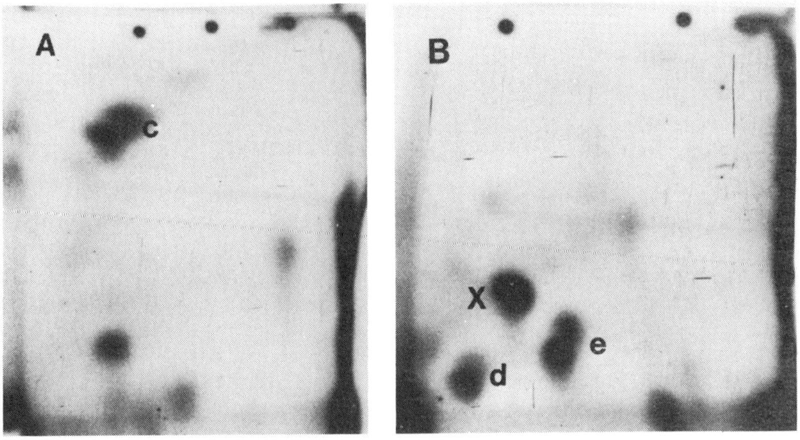

FIGURE 3. Autoradiograms of TLCs from a Saka villager in the first (A) and second (B) sampling of blood. The "X" spot, common in most individuals, and the sampling time specific spots "c", "d" and "e" are indicated. The sampling time specific spots were seen in most individuals studied.

Several alternatives exist to explain the differences noted. As the first it was noted that the villagers mainly lived in private houses with an own heating system, operated by peat and wood. Both the shale workers and the Tallinn controls lived mainly in apartment houses. As one explanation it was tested whether the villagers who lived in private houses (n=12) differed in the adduct levels from those living in apartment houses (n=4). Only a very minor difference was noted.

Another difference between the villages and the other populations was that all the villages had an own garden, which provided them produce as an important food supplement. In fact, all the villagers reported using their own produce as food. Thus it is not excluded that the differences noted would be related to environmental pollution contaminating the produce.

The presence of adducts is not unique to humans. When calf thymus DNA is postlabeled, many spots are seen in autoradiograms (Figure 4). The main spot appears similar to the "X"-spot seen in human samples.

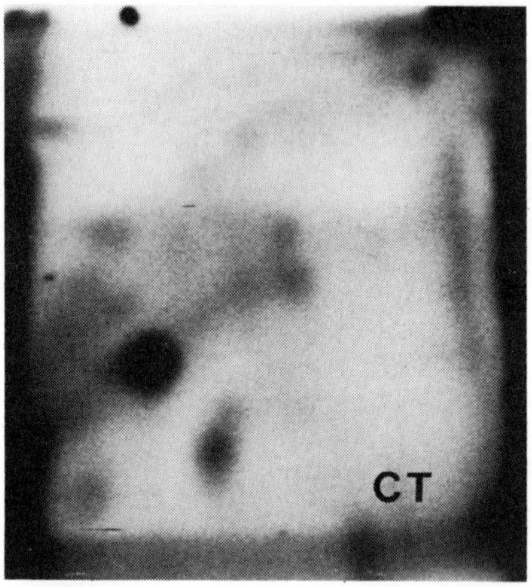

FIGURE 4. Calf thymus (= CT) DNA, digested and postlabeled as human DNA, shows a radioactive main spot similar to the "X" spot and many other minor spots of radioactivity.

Discussion

We showed here that some standard compounds, applicable to dietary studies, N-7-methyl-dGMP and the cyclic N1-N^2-dGMP derivatives of 4-hydroxy-2-nonenal are effectively labeled by T4 polynucleotide kinase. In addition to 4-hydroxy-2-nonenal, malonaldehyde adducts would be of interest as markers of lipid peroxidation[1,2,4,11].

In mice fed diet containing saturated fats and polysaturated fats, differences were observed in thiobarbituric acid-reactive compounds, such as malonaldehyde[26]. A similar difference was also noted in N-terminal valine adducts of reduced malonaldehyde in hemoglobin. The difference was increased by inducing lipid peroxidation by carbon tetrachloride. As hemoglobin adducts usually correlate with DNA adducts it is possible that differences could also be seen in DNA adducts.

The studies in healthy humans showed N-7-methyl-dGMP levels of 2.4 per 10^7 nucleotides, which was some 20 times less than that noted in patients treated with procarbazine and dacarbazine. In peripheral lung tissue of smokers the levels of N-7-methyl-dGMP have been measured at 10-50/10^7 nucleotides[23]. The source of N-7-methyl-dGMP in DNA remains unknown in untreated human DNA. The contribution by N-nitrosocompounds cannot be exclused[29,30].

In all human populations aromatic or polyaromatic (judged by chromatographic behaviour) can be detected at levels 1 adducts per 10^7 nucleotides[16,17]. As this is a total of all adducts found in the thin-layer plates, it suggests that any particular adduct is far less abundant than N-7-methyl-dGMP, assuming an equal labeling efficiency and recovery.

The origin of the adducts detected in healthy individuals is unknown. The most prominent adduct, the "X" spot, has been noted in almost all human and animal samples[18,19] but not at an equal intensity. The source of this adduct is unknown. Interestingly, calf thymus DNA showed adducts levels quite similar to control humans, including the apparent "X" spot. There are many uncertainties about human adduct studies, including classes of the adducts studied, their labeling efficiency, and, particularly, their origin[5,6,12,27]. It will be a long but exciting path to sort out these questions.

References

1 Bartsch H. The role of cyclic nucleic acid base adducts in carcinogenesis and mutagenesis. In: The role of cyclic nucleic acid base adducts in carcinogenesis and mutagenesis, ed B Singer, H Bartsch. Lyon: IARC Sci Publ 1986;70:3–14.

2 Chung F-L, Hecht SS, Palladino G. Formation of cyclic nucleic acid adducts from some simple α-unsaturated carbonyl compounds and cyclic nitrosamines. In: The role of cyclic nucleic acid base adducts in carcinogenesis and mutagenesis, ed B Singer, H Bartsch. Lyon: IARC Sci Publ 1986;70:207–25.

3 Doll R, Peto R. The causes of cancer: quantitative estimates of avoidable risks of cancer in the United States today. J Natl Cancer Inst 1981;66:1–73.

4 Esterbauer H. Aldehydic products of lipid peroxidation. In: Free Radicals, Lipid Peroxidation and Cancer, ed. DCH McBrien, TF Slater. London: Academic Press 1982:101–28.

5 Farmer PB, Neumann H-G, Henschler D. Estimation of exposure of man to substances reacting covalently with macromolecules. Arch Toxicol 1987;60:251–60.

6 Gorelick NJ, Wogan GN. Fluoranthene-DNA adducts: identification and quantification by an HPLC-^{32}P-postlabeling method. Carcinogenesis 1989;10:1567–77.

7 Gupta RC, Reddy MV, Randerath K. ^{32}P-postlabeling analysis of non-radioactive aromatic carcinogen-DNA adducts. Carcinogenesis 1982;3:1081–92.

8 Hemminki K, Peltonen K, Mustonen R. ^{32}P-postlabeling of 7-methyl-dGMP, ring-opened-dGMP and platinated dGdG. Chem-Biol Interact 1990;74:45–54.

9 Hemminki K, Szyfter K, Kadlubar FF. Quantitation of the ^{32}P-postlabeling reaction using N^1, N^2 and C8 modified deoxyguanosine 3'-monophosphates as substrates. Chem-Biol Interact 1990;76:51–61.

10 Hemminki K, Reunanen A, Kahn H. Use of DNA adducts in the assessment of occupational and environmental exposure to carcinogens. Eur J Cancer 1991 (in press).

11 Kautiainen A, Törnqvist M, Svensson K, Osterman-Golkar S. Adducts of malonaldehyde and a few other aldehydes to hemoglobin. Carcinogenesis 1989;10:2123–30.

12 Koivisto P, Hemminki K. ^{32}P-postlabeling of 2-hydroxyethylated, ethylated and methylated adduct of 2'-deoxyguanosine 3'-monophosphate. Carcinogenesis 1990;11:1389–92.

13 Miller AB (ed). Diet and the aetiology of cancer. ESO monographs. Berlin: Springer Verlag 1989:1-73.

14 Mustonen R, Hemminki K. Application of the ^{32}P-postlabeling technique to detect DNA-adducts by cisplatin and methylating agents. In: Mutation and the Environment, part C. Wiley-Liss, Inc. 1990:293–300.
15 Mustonen R, Hietanen P, Hemminki K, Measurement by ^{32}P-postlabeling of 7-methylguanine levels in white blood cell DNA of healthy individuals and cancer patients treated with dacarbazine and procarbazine. Carcinogenesis 1991 (in press).
16 Perera FP, Jeffrey A. Brandt-Rauf PW, Brenner D, Mayer JL, Smith SJ, Latriano L, Hemminki K, Santella RM. Molecular epidemiology and cancer prevention. Cancer Detect Prev 1990;14:639–45.
17 Perera FP, Mayer J, Santella RM, Brenner D, Jeffrey A, Latriano L, Smith S, Warburton D, Young TL, Tsai WY, Hemminki K, Brandt-Rauf PW. Biologic markers in risk assessment for environmental carcinogens. Environ Health Persp 1990:89.
18 Phillips DH, Hewer A, Martin CN, Garner RC, King MM. Correlation of DNA adduct levels in human lung with cigarette smoking. Nature 1988;336:790–2.
19 Phillips DH, Hemminki K, Alhonen A, Hewer A, Grover PL. Monitoring occupational exposure to carcinogens: detection by ^{32}P-postlabeling of aromatic DNA adducts in white blood cells from iron foundry workers. Mutat Res 1988;204:531–41.
20 Randerath K, Reddy MV, Gupta RC. ^{32}P-labeling test for DNA damage. Proc Natl Acad Sci USA 1981;78:6126–9.
21 Randerath K, Randerath E, Agraval HP, Gupta RC, Schurdak ME, Reddy MV. Postlabeling methods for carcinogen-DNA adduct analysis. Environ Health Persp 1985;62:57–65.
22 Reddy MV, Randerath K. Nuclease P1-mediated enhancement of sensitivity of ^{32}P-postlabeling test for structurally diverse DNA adducts. Carcinogenesis 1986;7:1531–43.
23 Shields PG, Povey AC, Wilson VL, Weston A, Harris CC. Combined high-performance liquid chromatography/^{32}P-postlabeling assay of N-7-methyldeoxyguanosine. Cancer Res 1990;50:6580–4.
24 Sodum RS, Chung F-L. 1,N^2-ethenodeoxyguanosine as a potential marker for DNA adduct formation by trans-4-hydroxy-2-nonenal. Cancer Res 1988;48:320–3.
25 Sodum RS, Chung F-L. Structural characterization of adducts formed in the reaction of 2,3-epoxy-4-hydroxynonanal with deoxyguanosine. Chem Rese Toxicol 1989;2:23–8.
26 Törnqvist M, Kautiainen A, Vaca CE, Anderstam B. In vivo hemoglobin-dosimetry of malonaldehyde and ethene in mice after induction of lipid peroxidation. Effects of membrane lipid fatty acid composition. Carcinogenesis 1991 (in press).
27 Vodicka P, Hemminki K. ^{32}P-postlabeling of N-7, N^2 and O^6 2'-deoxyguanosine 3'-monophosphate adducts of styrene oxide. Chem-Biol Interact 1990;76:39–50.
28 World Health Organization. Air quality guidelines for Europe. Copenhagen: World Health Organization 1987:105–17.
29 Wilson VL, Basu AK, Essigman JM, Smith RA, Harris CC. O-6-Alkyldeoxyguanosine detection by ^{32}P-postlabeling and nucleotider chromatographic analysis. Cancer Res 1988;48:2156–61.
30 Wilson VL, Weston A, Manchester DK, Trivers GE, Roberts DW, Kadlubar FF, Wild CP, Montesano R, Willey JC, Mann DL, Harris CC. Alkyl and aryl carcinogen adducts detected in human peripheral lung. Carcinogenesis 1989;10:2149–53.

8

Biomarkers for the apolipoprotein B gene, a candidate gene for atherosclerosis

MATTI J TIKKANEN

First Department of Medicine, Helsinki University Central Hospital, Helsinki, Finland

Introduction

Genetic factors have a major role in the etiology of atherosclerotic disorders. A number of studies have indicated this by demonstrating familial aggregation of these disorders, particularly of premature coronary heart disease (CHD)[2]. In addition to a family history positive for early CHD, elevated serum cholesterol is a major risk factor for CHD. Cholesterol levels may be influenced by genetic factors but they are also affected by environmental ones, such as diet, sex hormone status or sedentary life-style. Moreover, environmental factors may interact with genetic factors. For example, the differences in average serum cholesterol levels between apolipoprotein E (apoE) phenotypes are greater during a high-fat, high cholesterol diet than during a low-fat, low-cholesterol diet (Table 1)[11]. This is an example of the common phenomenon called gene-environment interaction (Figure 1).

While gene-environment interaction evidently is important in the etiology and pathogenesis of CHD, relatively little is known about the genes involved. The exploration of genetic factors contributing to development of "common" or "polygenic" hypercholesterolemia appears particularly important. The questions are: How can we identify the gene mutations or polymorphisms

Biomarkers of dietary exposure. Ed. F. J. Kok & P. van 't Veer.

TABLE 1. Total plasma cholesterol concentrations and changes during dietary study

Diet	E4/E4 (n=8)	E4/E3 (n=42)	E3/E3 (n=48)	E3/E2 (n=12)	ANOVA
High-fat, high-cholesterol diet	7.63	6.31	6.07	5.86	0.003
Low-fat, low-cholesterol diet	5.79	5.12	4.99	4.73	0.069
Switchback to high-cholesterol diet	7.31	6.00	5.99	5.53	0.002

Values are in mmol/l and are the means ± SD (ref. 11).

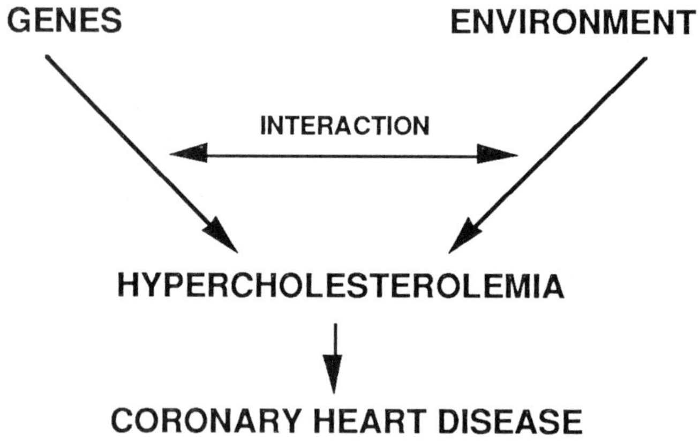

FIGURE 1. Gene-environment interaction

contributing to hypercholesterolemia. What are the gene-environment interactions involved. How can we benefit from knowing these mechanisms.

The candidate gene approach

For the clarification of the genetic basis of any disorder, a possible approach is to study those genes which according to the knowledge available seem to be most likely to be involved in the disease process. For example, the LDL-receptor gene regulating LDL-cholesterol uptake in the liver, and the HMG CoA reductase gene regulating cellular cholesterol synthesis would appear to be "candidate genes" for hypercholesterolemia. In their famous studies, Brown and Goldstein demonstrated that a number of mutations in the LDL-receptor gene resulted in familial hypercholesterolemia, a disorder characterized by severe hypercholesterolemia and premature CHD[3]. While this provides an example of the candidate gene concept it explains only a very small fraction of hypercholesterolemia. Thus other genes are probably involved in the development of the more common forms of this lipid disorder. From a theoretical point of view, a variety of genes coding for apolipoproteins, lipid metabolic enzymes, lipid transfer proteins, among others, can be regarded as potential candidate genes. However, the apolipoprotein B (apoB) gene is of particular interest, ApoB is the sole protein component of LDL and contains the binding site for the LDL-receptor, suggesting that mutant or polymorphic forms could interfere with the metabolic fate of LDL. The following account summarizes possible approaches to clarifying the role of the apoB gene changes in the etiology of hypercholesterolemia.

The apolipoprotein B gene

The first question is: are there mutant or polymorphic forms of apoB associated with hypercholesterolemia or other lipid disorders. If so, how can we identify these DNA changes. In exploring these questions one may consider the following 5-step approach. The sequence of the steps depends on whether one is looking for causes of common hypercholesterolemia or rare mutations. For commonly occurring variants, one may start the sequence from step 1. The search for rare mutations may start from detection of a functional deficiency (step 4), followed by family studies and identification of the causative DNA sequence change. The latter approach is exemplified by the clarification of the mutation causing *familial defective apoB-100*, the first apoB ligand defect shown to cause hypercholesterolemia (see below)[7].

1. Identification of genetic markers

The first markers used for the apoB gene were epitopes for monospecific antibodies (*protein* markers). Currently a variety of restriction fragment length polymorphism (RFLP) alleles and hypervariable region (HVR) alleles (*DNA* markers) are being utilized. While the protein markers always indicate an amino acid change, many DNA markers are base changes which do not result in any change in the protein itself (e.g. apoB XbaI or HVR alleles). The importance of the "silent" DNA markers lies in their possible linkage with functionally important (causative) mutations. Multiallelic markers (HVR alleles) are superior to biallelic markers (RFLP alleles) in segregation analyses. Combination of several markers of the same gene provides the opportunity to use haplotypes in family studies. Some of the recently studied protein and DNA markers of the apoB gene will be discussed in the following section.

2. Search for population associations

Monoclonal anti-apoB antibodies are currently being used for detecting epitopes previously defined by Ag antisera. For example, the Ag(c/g) polymorphism can be studied by antibody MB-19. When this antibody was used to study 513 Finnish 9-year-old children the results indicated that the Ag(c) allele was associated with a slightly but significantly higher serum cholesterol and apoB level than the Ag(g) allele[10]. Studies in adult populations using similar methodology did not detect this association. We speculated that this weak association became detectable in the child population because of its homogeneity (same age and ethnic origin), and because the variation caused by environmental factors (diet, life-style differences) was minimized. The XbaI RFLP of the apoB gene has become the most widely studied polymorphism because the X2 allele (cutting site present) was shown to be associated with higher serum cholesterol than the X1 allele (cutting site absent) in some populations, including the Finns. However, the association has not been confirmed in all populations studied. The Ag(c) and X2 alleles were shown to be in linkage disequilibrium[5] and the combined genotype [X2 and Ag(c) alleles present] was associated with higher cholesterol than either allele alone in Finnish individuals[1] (Figure 2).

ASSOCIATIONS WITH APO B GENETIC MARKERS

POLYMORPHISM	MARKERS	PHENOTYPE
apo B Xbal	X2 allele	cholesterol ↑
apo B c/g	c allele	cholesterol ↑

X2 vs c: linkage disequilibrium ($p<0.01$)

FIGURE 2.

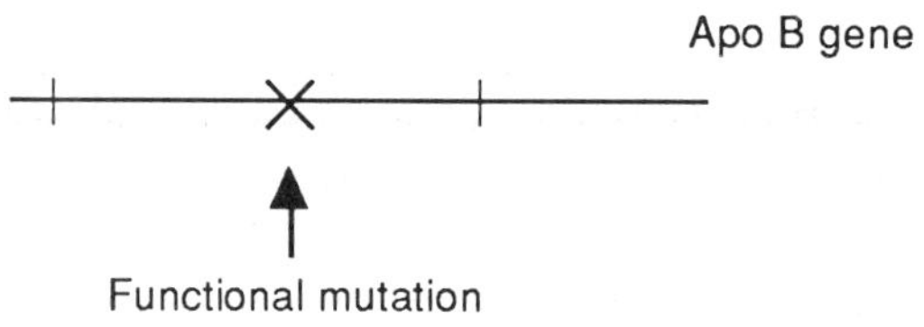

FIGURE 3. Hypothesis: The XbaI and c/g polymorphic sites are probably in linkage disequilibrium with a yet unknown functionally important mutation. The positioning of the hypothetical functional mutation in relation to the two polymorphic sites is arbitrary.

The results from these population studies suggested that there were alterations in the apoB gene causing differences in serum cholesterol. However, the markers used were only weakly associated with cholesterol levels and the associations were not observed in all populations. Our hypothesis is that both markers are in linkage disequilibrium with a yet unknown causative DNA change (Figure 3).

3. Family studies

Any significant population association can be further analyzed by studying the possible co-segregation of marker and cholesterol elevation in families. It should be pointed out that population studies cannot be replaced by family studies. Relatively small average effects, such as those exerted by apoE alleles on serum cholesterol, could not have been detected in family studies. In line with this, family studies have not been helpful with the Ag(c) or XbaI X2 allele studies, because of the weak average effects of these alleles on serum cholesterol, and because of the variation caused by numerous environmental factors. Conversely, rare mutations (e.g. LDL-receptor defects) are difficult to detect in population association studies but co-segregation of mutation and phenotype (e.g. LDL-receptor defect and high cholesterol) is easily demonstrable in kindreds.

4. Characterization of mutant allele with respect to function

The LDL-receptor binding affinity of low density lipoprotein particles isolated from individuals with a certain marker (e.g. the apoB X2 allele) may be assayed in fibroblast cultures[8], or the clearance of radiolabelled LDL from the circulation can be assessed in turnover studies[4]. The association between an apoB marker and a functional deficiency (impaired receptor binding or clearance) would then indicate the involvement of the apoB gene. This could, for example, result from a yet unknown DNA sequence change in linkage with the marker. This DNA change could presumably be located in the region coding for the receptor bindings site, or for some other part of the protein which influences its metabolic fate.

5. Identification of functionally important DNA changes

The approach presented in the previous section is exemplified by the discovery of the first apoB mutation causing hypercholesterolemia, the disorder called *familial defective apoB-100*[7]. The mutation results in the glutamine-for-arginine substitution at amino acid residue 3500. The functional deficiency was initially detected in turnover studies in which certain patients expressed a reduced capacity to clear autologous radiolabelled LDL from their circulation but were able to normally clear heterologous LDL[13]. This indicated that the patients had normal LDL-receptor function and suggested that their LDL contained defective apoB. Further studies using fibroblast cultures confirmed that the LDL isolated from these patients expressed reduced binding to the LDL-receptor, a monoclonal antibody (MB-47) was shown to react differently with the apoB from the patients suggesting the possibility that the causative DNA change could reside in the DNA region coding for the MB-47 epitope[14]. Sequencing of the DNA region coding for the amino acid sequences involved in the receptor binding site and MB-47 epitope revealed only one unique mutation in codon 3500[9].

Discussion

The current knowledge concerning the role of the apoB gene in hypercholesterolemia may be summarized as follows. We know that some commons biallelic variations (e.g. XbaI and Ag(c/g) polymorphisms) are associated with altered serum cholesterol levels. This suggests the existence of at least one common polymorphic DNA change which causes a functionally important alteration in the apoB protein and results in cholesterol elevation. The markers discussed above are probably in linkage disequilibrium with this DNA sequence change which has resulted in significant associations between markers and serum cholesterol. At this writing, sequencing efforts have failed to identify the relevant DNA change.

With regard to less common polymorphisms and rare mutations, only one functionally important apoB amino acid change has been described. This is the substitution of glutamine for arginine at amino acid residue 3500 causing familial defective apoB-100. According to one estimate, based on screening of 1100 individuals in North America and Austria, the frequency of this disorder would be 1:500[7]. In Finland the screening of 552 hypercholesterolemic subjects did not reveal a single case[6] suggesting a markedly lower frequency. The exploration for other mutations affecting the binding of apoB to receptors, or other metabolic events, is now being pursued by many laboratories by searching for functionally deficient LDL in hypercholesterolemic kindreds.

The studies on the apoB gene and other candidate genes form the basis for the elucidation of the genetic architecture of hypercholesterolemia. While this constitutes only a part of the genetic architecture of CHD, it may be worthwhile to define genotypes causing susceptibility to cholesterol-elevating environmental factors. As genotypes are unalterable, CHD prevention strategies must be based minimizing adverse gene-environment interactions. There is already preliminary evidence from diet intervention studies indicating that cholesterol-elevating effects of certain genotypes can be ameliorated by dietary modification[11,12].

References

1 Aalto-Setälä K, Tikkanen MJ, Taskinen M-R, et al. XbaI and c/g polymorphisms of the apolipoprotein B gene locus are associated with serum cholesterol and LDL-cholesterol levels in Finland. Atherosclerosis 1988;74:47–54.

2 Berg K. Genetics of coronary heart disease. In: eds AG Steinberg et al Prog Med Genet. Philadelphia: WB Saunders Co 1983: Vol V:35–90.
3 Brown MS, Goldstein J. A receptor-mediated pathway for cholesterol homeostasis. Science 1986;232:34–47.
4 Demant T, Houlston RS, Caslake MJ, et al. Catabolic rate of low density lipoprotein is influenced by variation in the apolipoprotein B gene. J Clin Invest 1988;82:797–802.
5 Dunning AM, Tikkanen MJ, Ehnholm C, Butler R, Humphries SE. Relationships between DNA and protein polymorphisms of apolipoprotein B. Human Genet 1988;78:325–9.
6 Hämäläinen T, Palotie A, Aalto-Setätä K, et al. Asence of familial defective apoB-100 in Finnish patients with elevated plasma cholesterol. Atherosclerosis 1990;82:177–83.
7 Innerarity TL, Mahley RW, Weisgraber KH, et al. Familial defective apolipoprotein B-100: a mutation of apolipoprotein B that causes hypercholesterolemia. J Lipid Res 1990;31:1337–49.
8 Series J, Cameron I, Caslake M, et al. The XbaI polymorphism of the apolipoprotein B gene influences the degradation of low density lipoprotein in vitro. Biochim Biophys Acta 1989;1003:183–8.
9 Soria LF, Ludwig E, Clarke HRG, et al. Association between a specific apolipoprotein B mutation and familial defective apolipoprotein B-100. Proc Natl Acad Sci USA 1989;86:587–91.
10 Tikkanen MJ. Viikari J. Åkerblom H. Pesonen E. Apolipoprotein B polymorphism associated with altered apolipoprotein B and low-density lipoprotein levels in Finnish children. Br Med J 1988;296:169–70.
11 Tikkanen MJ, Huttunen JK, Ehnholm C, Pietinen P. Apolipoprotein E4 homozygosity predisposes to serum cholesterol elevation during high fat diet. Arteriosclerosis 1990;10:285–8.
12 Tikkanen MJ. Xu C-F, Hämäläinen T, et al. XbaI polymorphism of the apolipoprotein B gene influences plasma lipid response to diet intervention. Clin Genet 1990;37:327–34.
13 Vega GL, Grundy SM. In vivo evidence for reduced binding of low density lipoproteins to receptors as a cause of primary moderate hypercholesterolemia. J Clin Invest 1986;78:1410–4.
14 Weisgraber KH, Innerarity TL, Newhouse Y, et al. Familial defective apolipoprotein B-100: enhanced binding of monoclonal antinody MB-47 to abnormal low density lipoproteins. Proc Natl Acad Sci USA 1988;85:9758–62.

9

Workshop I: Energy

Energy expenditure as a biomarker of energy intake: workshop report
SHEILA A. BINGHAM and KLAAS R WESTERTERP

Validations of dietary assessment using doubly labelled water
A.E. BLACK et al.

Accuracy of energy intake measurements in 3–18 year old subjects
M.B.E. LIVINGSTONE et al.

Body composition as a biomarker of nutritional and physical development status
J. PARÍZKOVÁ

Are available reference growth data and recommendations for energy intake still appropriate for evaluation of present-day energy intake in infancy?
M. KERSTING et al.

Evaluating dietary surveys against energy requirements
A.E. BLACK et al.

Validation of the 7-day weighed record and the dietary history by 24-hour energy expenditure measurements in a whole body calorimeter
L.C.P.G.M. de GROOT et al.

Assessment of energy intake and physical activity: an evaluation of dietary records, activity records and an accelerometer against doubly labelled water
K.R. WESTERTERP et al.

Biomarkers of dietary exposure. Ed. F. J. Kok & P. van 't Veer.

Energy expenditure as a biomarker of energy intake: workshop report

SHEILA A. BINGHAM and KLAAS R. WESTERTERP

Dunn Clinical Nutrition Centre Cambridge, United Kingdom; Department of Human Biology, University of Limburg, Maastricht, Netherlands

Doubly labelled water is accepted as an accurate method of measuring total energy expenditure, provided that well established procedures are followed. Problems with fractionation, repeatability, interlaboratory comparisons were discussed, but these have been extensively considered elsewhere[1]. It was agreed that on a group basis, total energy expenditure can be estimated from Basal Metabolic Rate (BMR), assuming values published by WHO, which are supported by more recent field and calorimetry data. There was also consensus that the ratio of energy intake to estimated BMR is acceptable as a useful measure of the validity of assessments of dietary intake. There have been new non-invasive developments in monitoring physical activity for the estimation of total energy expenditure. This is more accurate for predicting energy expenditure than estimates from BMR only, but less expensive and technologically easier than $^{2}H_{2}\,^{18}O$. It was unanimously accepted that underreporting of energy intake has been shown to occur when compared with these measures of energy expenditure, in otherwise weight stable subjects. This is a consistent finding in obese adults and seems more likely in females. There is too little data to attribute underreporting to a specific dietary survey method.

Ideally BMR should be individually and directly measured by standard techniques. However, equations for predicting BMR from body weight and height exist[2] and these are reliable (± 10% for individuals of normal weight (Body Mass Index: 20-25 kg/m). Uncertainties at the extremes of body weight exist, and more data are needed, with full reports of experimental conditions.

More validations with whole body calorimetry of the $^{2}H_{2}\,^{18}O$ technique in obese subjects were suggested. Other means of obtaining total energy intake are required, but questionnaires used to assess activity level are generally inaccurate. Reliable activity monitors exist, but need to be marketed.

Underreporting on a group basis has been described, but it is not clear whether all individuals within the population underreport by a similar amount, or whether a sub-group is responsible. If so, how can this be characterised by different methods for measuring energy expenditure, and should intake results from this group be treated separately? The reasons for underreporting need to be established. Is this due to slimming, is it intentional, or is it unintentional? New ways for assessing this are needed. Is it a particular food, or group of foods that is underreported? What effect does underreporting of energy have on intakes of other nutrients? This could be assessed perhaps with other biological markers.

Since the validity of different dietary survey techniques seem to vary between different populations, it is not acceptable to rely on literature reports of the accuracy of a particular technique. A minimal requirement is that all new studies need to demonstrate the extent to which energy intake agrees with energy expenditure at the group level. Future studies should therefore repeat data on age, sex, height, and weight. Ideally weight changes should be monitored over the observation period.

Direct practical applications in the field of analytic and descriptive epidemiology are to assess validity of dietary methodology regarding energy intake. On a group level the BMR ratio should be between 1.5 to 2.1[3]. For individual assessment the acceptable BMR ratio is uncertain, but habitual values below 1.2 are not realistic. Finally, in intervention studies the implied changes in energy intake should be validated, ideally with $^{2}H_{2}\,^{18}O$, or alternatively by activity monitoring.

References

1 International Dietary Energy Consultancy Group. The doubly labelled water method for measuring energy expenditure. Prentice AM. ed. International Atomic Energy Authority, Vienna 1990.

2 Schofield WN, Schofield C, James WPT. Basal metabolic rate. Human Nutr: Clin Nutr 1985;39C,Suppl.1:1–96.

3 World Health Organisation Energy and protein requirements. Tech. Rep. Ser. 724, WHO, Geneva. 1985.

Validations of dietary assessment using doubly labelled water*

A.E. BLACK, G.R. GOLDBERG, S.A. JEBB, S.A. BINGHAM, M.B.E. LIVINGSTONE and AM PRENTICE

Dunn Clinical Nutrition Centre, Cambridge, United Kingdom

Daily variation in food intake means that few dietary assessments measure the true mean food intake of individuals, but random sampling should result in a valid measure of the long-term mean ("habitual") intake of the group. Most studies of diet and health make the tacit assumption that either a valid measure of "habitual" food intake is obtained, or that bias, if present, operates equally across all subjects and thus within study comparisons remain valid. Only independent external markers of intake can verify these assumptions.

In a weight stable population Energy Intake (EI) must equal Energy Expenditure (EE). Free-living EE can be measured by the Doubly Labelled Water technique (DLW) which can thus be used as external validation of EI. Results from studies in which we have measured both EE and EI are presented.

Study		Method	EE J/d	EI MJ/d	EI:EEI Mean	sd (range)
Black et al. in prep.	7 students volunteers	10d WI1	10.50	10.70	1.02	0.13 (0.84–1.18)
		10d WI2	11.16	10.59	0.96	0.10 (0.82–1.05)
Prentice et al.[4] and unpublished	15 lean women volunteers	7d WI	8.44	7.97	0.96	0.17 (0.63–1.14)
Goldberg et al.[2]	10 lean women volunteers	7d WI	9.7	9.42	0.98	0.17 (0.69–1.30)
Livingstone et al.[3]	16 men R	7d WI	14.23	11.21	0.81	0.22 (0.46–1.40)
	15 women R	7d WI	9.93	8.00	0.82	0.21 (0.45–1.18)
Black et al.[1]	11 postobese volunteers	10d WI	9.73	6.66	0.74	0.17 (0.47–0.95)
		106 PT	9.73	7.22	0.79	0.22 (0.46–1.14)
		DHA	9.57	6.61	0.64	0.20 (0.38–0.98)
		DHB	9.57	7.66	0.84	0.21 (0.55–1.15)
Prentice et al.[4]	9 obese women volunteers	2x7d WI	10.22	6.73	0.64	0.17 (0.38–0.87)

R=part of a random sample
WI=Weighed records, PT=weighed records PETRA system, DH=diet history.

Lean subjects never overweight volunteering for a demanding project showed good agreement between EI and EE; a subsample of a randomly selected population showed less good agreement suggesting poorer motivation to comply with study demands; obese and postobese showed poor agreement, confirming suspicions that these subjects misrepresent their intake. Further work is needed to quantify errors and identify poor compliers.

References

1 Black et al. Proc Nutr Soc 1991 (in press).
2 Goldberg et al. Proc Nutr Soc 1991 (in press).
3 Livingstone et al. Br Med J 1990;300:708–12.
4 Prentice et al. Br Med J 1986;292:983–87.

* Presented at plenary session

Accuracy of energy intake measurements in 3–18 year old subjects

M.B.E. LIVINGSTONE[1], A.M. PRENTICE[2], P.S.W. DAVIES[2], A.E. BLACK[2], W.A. COWARD[2], C. STEWART[1] and J.J. STRAIN[1]

[1]Biomedical Sciences Research Centre, University of Ulster and [2]MRC Dunn Nutrition Unit, Cambridge, United Kingdom

Food intakes of children and adolescents were independently evaluated by comparison with measured energy expenditure. Energy intakes (EI) were assessed by 7-day weighed dietary record (WDR) and by diet history (DH) in 78 subjects aged 3, 5, 7, 9, 12, 15 and 18 years. (41 males, 37 females). WDR were not obtained from the 3 and 5 year olds. The results were compared with concurrent estimates of total energy expenditure (TEE) by the doubly-labelled water method.

Age (years)		3	5	7	9	12	15	18
n		8	12	12	12	12	12	10
TEE (MJ/d)	Mean	5.26	6.09	7.62	8.78	10.54	11.71	13.50
	SD	0.68	1.26	1.38	1.26	1.10	2.77	4.11
DH (MJ/d)	Mean	5.91*	6.55	8.48*	9.28*	11.96*	11.62	12.83
	SD	0.55	0.71	1.62	1.19	2.02	3.04	3.38
WDR (MJ/d)	Mean	–	–	8.19	8.45	9.36**	9.08**	9.28**
	SD	2.16	1.36	1.54	2.92	3.00		

Significantly different from TEE value (paired t test): * $p < 0.05$, ** $p < 0.01$

The younger children (7 and 9 years) appeared to provide reliable record of EI by WDR but in adolescents (n = 34) EI was substantially underestimated, particularly by girls ($p < 0.001$). The bias was > 20% in 13 adolescents and reached 50% in 5 subjects. In contrast no age or gender specific trend in misreporting was apparent in EI assessed by DH. These results suggest that the WDR is prone to biased under-reporting of food intake in adolescents, particularly the girls. The DH is more reliable at the level of group comparisons but inconsistencies in dietary reporting at the individual level highlight the problem of applying this methodology to children.

This study was supported by the Department of Health, UK

Body composition as a biomarker of nutritional and physical development status

J. PARIZKOVÁ

Research Institute for Physical Education, Charles University, Prague, Czechoslovakia

Body composition (lean body mass and depot fat in absolute and relative quantities) is widely used during the whole life span as a biomarker of the nutritional status and balance between energy intake and output. The latter is mostly due to the amount and character of physical activity and/or work load. Therefore, body composition characterizes at the same time also then level of physical activity and fitness. Adequate nutritional and physicals performance status may not always run parallel: the analysis of the mutual relationships of the abovementioned items gives more accurate information/on physical development status.

The amount of body fat as measured by a number of methods correlates significantly with the level of triglycerides and cholesterol in the serum and with body mass index, as well as a number of other functional and metabolic parameters, starting with preschool age. In the range of usual values of food intake (i.e. excluding starving) no correlation was found between body fat and energy, and/or individual food items intake in preschool and adult subjects.

In the obese, body composition was the best marker of the results of the reduction therapy, showing approximately also the composition of weight decrements.

Are available reference growth data and recommendations for energy intake still appropriate for evaluation of present-day energy intake in infancy?

M. KERSTING, E. MAUBNER, A. KORFMANN and G. SCHÖCH

Forschungsinstitut für Kinderernährung, Dortmund, Germany

Problem

Growth is a sensitive and at the same time easily available indicator of the adequacy of energy intake in infancy. From results of recent, but only sporadic, longitudinal growth and nutrition studies of infants, it has come into discussion, that the recommendations for energy intake might be too high and that reference growth data might be inappropriate for present-day infants. Two recent longitudinal nutrition and growth studies during the first year of life of infants in Dortmund support these discussions.

Methods

Study 1: 1987–1988, 38 infants, highly-motivated mothers, intensive nutrition counselling, infant nutrition according closely to pediatric recommendations (exclusive breast-feeding (60%) or partially breast-feeding/adapted formula (40%) during months 1–4, introduction of "beikost" meals gradually during months 5–7). Nutrition survey: precise-weighing-method in monthly intervals. Study 2: 1986–1989, random subsample of 120 infants from a representative sample of 708 infants, no dietary counselling (exclusive breast-feeding during months 1–4 only 18%, "beikost" for 42:51:75% of infants at the ends of months 2/3/4). Nutrition survey: 24hr-recall in monthly intervals, calculations of energy intake only possible for formula-fed infants. In both studies, weight and length measurements during visits at home at monthly intervals.

Results

Average energy intake (kcal/kg bodyweight/day) during months 1–12 in study 1 was 10–15% below recommendations (US-RDA, WHO) in study 2 almost in accordance with the recommendations. Growth status (median weight/height) in both studies was 105-110% of reference values (US-NCHS, UK-Tanner) until months 3–4, decreased until month 6 and remained near the reference values during months 7–12.

In the (only small) subsamples of breast-fed (> 3 months exclusively) or initially formula-fed infants in study 2, there seemed to be no consistent differences in growth status during the first year of life. The observation of a higher average energy intake of the infants in study 2 as compared to study 1 and study 2 will be discussed in the presentation (e.g. energy utilization from human milk higher than that from formula?, over(under)estimation of energy intake by recall (weighing)?). In both studies, abnormalities as to morbidity or behaviour of the infants have not been observed.

Conclusions

In accordance with the results of other authors, average energy intake below the current recommendations with an overall wellbalanced diet (study 1) does not seem to be detrimental to the health of infants. Current recommendations for energy intake and common reference growth data therefore might not be appropriate standards for present-day infants. However, more longitudinal growth and nutrition data are necessary to support the recently observed phenomena.

Evaluating dietary surveys against energy requirements

A.E. BLACK, G.R. GOLDBERG, S.A. JEBB and A.M. PRENTICE

Dunn Clinical Nutrition Centre, Cambridge, United Kingdom

There is a strong probability that dietary surveys under-estimate "habitual" food intake. This conclusion rests on considerations of energy physiology. FAO/WHO/UNU[1] expressed energy requirements as multiples of Basal Metabolic Rate. The average for a sedentary lifestyle is given as 1.55 × BMR. Since most dietary surveys also measure height and weight, mean BMR can be calculated from equations[2] and related to the reported mean energy intake (EI/BMR).

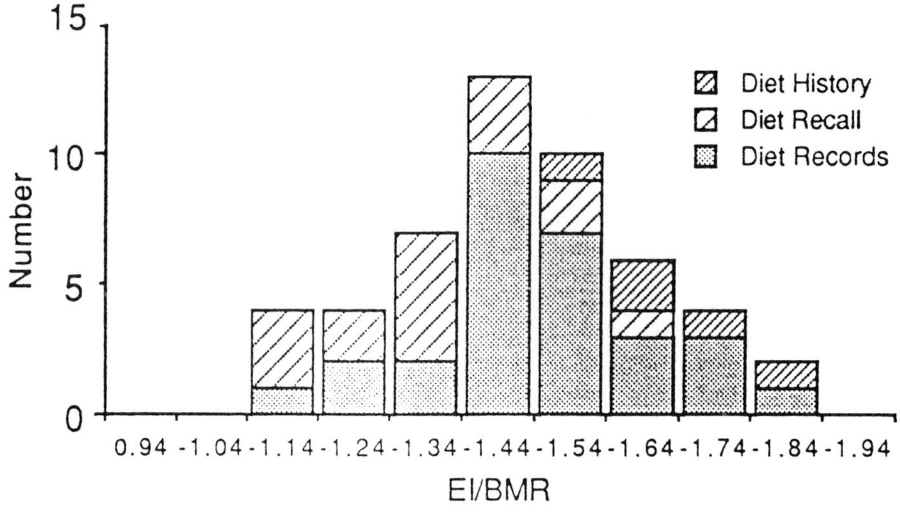

FIGURE 1. EI/BMR in published diet surveys of adults.

The figure shows the distribution of EI/BMR in 50 subgroups from 28 studies of adults in 8 countries of Europe and America ranging from n=10 to n=10,000 and including different survey methods. In only 12 groups does EI/BMR reach or exceed 1.55. It is statistically improbable for all intakes below 1.55 × BMR to be valid measures of "habitual" intake even for very sedentary lifestyles. Intakes above 1.55 × BMR could also be underestimations of intakes by more physically active groups. Survey method has an influence. Records, weighed or in household measures, give varied EI/BMR; Recall tends to give lower and History higher values. EI/BMR is higher for men

(1.49 ± 0.17) than woman (1.32 ± 0.17) indicating either better compliance or higher activity levels.

Evidence to indicate whether bias to underestimation is due to an observer effect operating equally on all subjects, or to subgroups who could be identified and excluded from analysis, or to a continuum of good to bad records is scanty. At present data has to be taken at face value while maintaining a critical awareness of possible misinterpretations.

References

1 FAO/WHO/UNU. Energy and protein requirements. Wld Health Org Techn Rep Ser 742. Geneva, 1985.
2 Schofield WN. Hum Nutr Clin Nutr 1985;39C Suppl.1:5–41.

Validation of the 7-day weighed record and the dietary history by 24-hour energy expenditure measurements in a whole body calorimeter

L.C.P.G.M. de GROOT, J.O. de BOER and W.A. van STAVEREN

Department of Human Nutrition, Agricultural University, Wageningen, The Netherlands

For energy intake no physiological measure of intake is available. Yet 24-hour energy expenditure (24EE) measurements can be used to validate dietary intake, assuming that both measurements are estimates of energy requirement. In two separate studies usual energy intake according to the 7-day weighed record and the dietary history was compared with 24-hour energy expenditure.

In 27 lean and 18 overweight woman (BMI 20.7 ± 1.9 and 33.5 ± 6.9 kg/m^2) energy intake was estimated by the 7-day weighed record. Energy intake of lean women (8.6 ± 1.7 MJ/d) was similar to 24EE (8.62 ± 0.73 MJ/d) and correlated positively ($r = 0.58$, $p < 0.005$). Therefore the 7-day weighed record seems to give valid estimates of the usual energy intake of lean women. In overweight women, however, a daily intake of on average 18% (1.9 ± 2.9 MJ/d) below 24EE (10.70 ± 1.91 MJ/d) was reported. Deviations from 24EE varied widely (up to –69%) and no significant association between intake and expenditure was found.

In a comparable study among 27 (moderately) obese women (BMI: 29.6 ± 4.5 kg/m^2) the group means of energy intake (9.6 ± 2.0 MJ/d) according to a dietary history (which tends to overestimate energy intake), agreed well with 24EE (9.80 ± 1.01 MJ/d). Within the group of overweight women underestimation of energy intake tends to increase with increasing BMI. This tendency was confirmed by a declining physical activity index with body weight. Due to the dependency of mean intakes on the weight distribution within the group of overweight women, the validity of the dietary history is questionable in this group.

Both studies illustrate the phenomenon of a non-constant bias related to obesity, even within a group of overweight women. This bias may hinder a ranking of overweight subjects according to their dietary intakes.

Assessment of energy intake and physical activity: an evaluation of dietary records, activity records and an accelerometer against doubly labelled water

K.R. WESTERTERP, D.L.E. PANNEMANS, G.A.L. MEIJER and W.H.M. SARIS

Department of Human Biology, University of Limburg, Maastricht, The Netherlands

In nutrition research, usually, food intake and physical activity in daily life are assessed by self report. The most reliable method is a 7-day record although this method may easily influence the behaviour of the subject. Less cumbersome but also less reliable are questionnaires about habitual physical activity. Nowadays, physical activity can also be monitored over weekly intervals using motion sensors. Energy expenditure in daily life can be accurately measured using doubly labelled water (DLW). Here we present a number of studies in which energy intake (EI) and physical activity (PA) were measured with a record (EI, PA), a questionnaire (PA), or an accelerometer (PA) developed in our institute. All assessments were carried out with simultaneous measurement of energy expenditure (EE) with DLW and resting metabolic rate (RMR) with respirometry.

Study	Subjects	EI	PA
1 Meijer et al.[1]	11 obese 11 lean	7-day record	7-day accelerometer
2 Westerterp et al.[3]	13 lean	7-day record (4-times)	questionnaire 7-day accelerometer
3 Pannemans et al.[2]	10 elderly	7-day record	questionnaire 7-day record

Subjects in all studies were weight stable over the observation intervals. In the first observation, reported EI in lean subjects was close to measured EE (EI–EE = 12 ± 17% of EE). In obese subjects, reported intake was too low (EI–EE = –26 ± 18% of EE). The extent of underreporting was closely related to the body mass index ($p < 0.001$).

Underreporting increased when subjects were observed more than once, 8–20 weeks afterwards ($p < 0.01$, study 2).

Physical activity measured with a 7–day record was related to the calculated PA (EE/RMR, $p < 0.05$), whereas with a standard questionnaire no relation was found (study 3). A motion sensor gave reliable information on PA, explaining 77% of the variation in the activity compartment of EE (study 1 + 2).

In conclusion, data on food intake and physical activity collected with questionnaires and records have to be interpreted with great care. A validation against DLW in a sample of the study population is needed. The accelerometer is a realistic alternative for weekly records to monitor physical activity.

References

1 Meijer GAL et al. Int J Obes 1991 (in press).
2 Pannemans et al. (in preparation).
3 Westerterp KR et al. Br J Nutr 1991 (in press).

10

Workshop II: Fatty acids

Biomarkers of fatty acids: workshop report
RUUD A. RIEMERSMA and LIISA M. VALSTA

Plasma fatty acid pattern as a biological marker for dietary intake of long chain n-3 fatty acids
C.A. DREVON et al.

Triglyceride pattern of human sera as marker for vegetarian nutrition
H.U. MELCHERT et al.

Potential use of magnetic resonance spectroscopy to monitor:compliance with taking fish oil supplements: a pilot study
P.C. DAGNELIE et al.

Effect of the short-term day-to-day variability of serum lipids on the accuracy of CHD-risk assignment
C. SCACCINI et al.

Variability in cholesterol and fatty acids intake in the south of Spain. Something to consider when a biomarkers study is planned
J. GÓMEZ-ARACENA et al.

Questionnaire and tissue measures of dietary fat intake in Jerusalem
J.D. KARK et al.

Polyunsaturated fatty acids in adipose tissue in 38-year old European men in relation to serum lipids, smoking habits, and fat distribution
J.C. SEIDELL et al.

The fatty acid composition of plasma fatty acids after diets high in rapeseed oil or sunflower oil
I. AHOLA et al.

Biomarkers of dietary exposure. Ed. F. J. Kok & P. van 't Veer.

Biomarkers of fatty acids: workshop report

RUUD A RIEMERSMA and LIISA M VALSTA

Cardiovascular Research Unit, University of Edinburgh, Scotland;
Department of Nutrition, University of Helsinki, Helsinki, Finland

There is increasing interest in the role of diet in the development and ultimately in the prevention of coronary heart disease on a community basis. Monitoring of diets using weighed dietary inventory methods is very time consuming and it is therefore not surprising that alternative approaches are taken. A novel method, using nuclear magnetic resonance spectroscopy (NMR) was developed to monitor compliance in subjects taking fish oil capsules in a pilot study (Dagnelie et al). The value of high resolution NMR is that it is now possible to identify specific signals in plasma. One of the advantages is that the chemical shift of these NMR signals, due to naturally abundant ^{13}C, differs between the dietary fatty acids and will allow the monitoring of the incorporation of individual fatty acids in plasma lipids. As yet this work is done in vitro, but ultimately it should be possible to make in vivo measurements, particularly if ^{13}C fish oils became available.

Two studies reported on dietary intake of polyunsaturated, monounsaturated and saturated fatty acids derived from food frequency questionnaire (Kark et al) and 48 hour recall, respectively (Gómez-Aracena et al).

The fat consumption in Israel increased from a low mean of 28% of energy 25 years ago to a current 36%, and the polyunsaturated/saturated fatty acid ratio remained high. Despite the increase in total fat consumption mortality from coronary heart disease declined over the last two decades. The dietary assessment was validated in this study by adipose tissue and red blood cell fatty acid analysis in 75% of a sample of the Jewish population of Jerusalem.

In the Spanish study, seasonal differences in polyunsaturated fatty acids were observed, with higher intake during the summer. Whether seasonal variations in plasma lipid fatty acid composition was measured is not clear, but these results suggest that these may well vary. Seasonal variations in adipose linoleate levels have not been observed in studies in Edinburgh (Riemersma et al, unpublished). The implications for short-term or long-term studies are obvious.

The fatty acids composition of serum phospholipids, cholesteryl esters and triglycerides were determined by gaschromatography to examine whether dietary alpha-linolenic acid (2 energy %) is efficiently converted to eicosapentaenoic acid (Ahola et al). Competition for incorporation into phospholipids between n-6 and n-3 fatty acids was assessed by comparing an alpha-linoleic acid rich diet with a diet rich in linolenic acid. It is concluded that the conversion of alpha-linolenic acid to eicosapentaenoic acid in man is very limited. A new method, combining argentation chromatography and reverse phase high performance liquid chromatography was developed to analyse triglyceride isomers (Melchert and Kemper). Distinctive patterns of triglycerides were observed in vegetarians and non-vegetarians.

Polyunsaturated fat diets reduce blood pressure and serum cholesterol. Seidell et al examined the relation between adipose polyunsaturated fatty acids and serum lipids, smoking and obesity in five European countries. Although the relation between adipose linoleic or alpha-linolenic and serum lipids differed between centres, analysis of the pooled data showed an inverse correlation between adipose linoleate and total or LDL cholesterol. A similar inverse relation exists between alpha-linolenate and serum triglycerides. These associations remained significant after adjusting for smoking and body mass indices. As has been observed before, these measurements explain relatively little of the variation in serum lipids. Nevertheless the authors conclude that long-term adipose fatty acid composition, reflecting long-term dietary habits, are related to lipid metabolism. The associations with blood pressure were not mentioned in this report.

The biological variability of serum lipids during a ten-day period was the subject of another study (Scaccini et al). The variability in fasting serum triglycerides was highest (17%) whilst that of total cholesterol and HDL cholesterol was less (both 5%) in young volunteers (< 40 years). In older subjects the variability tended to be less. Several measurements (up to 4) have to be made to accurately characterise the lipid profile of young individuals.

There was a lively discussion on the strengths and weaknesses of fatty acid composition as a reflection of dietary intake. Nevertheless, there was relatively little discussion from the nutritionists in the audience. The development of a new method to analyze triglyceride fatty acids composition was discussed. The method involving several steps (argentation and HPL chromatography) can easily be carried out by technicians. High temperature GLC cannot give as much detailed information as yet and there may be several problems (degradation etc.). The development of a fully automated system is feasible and also the development of chromatography columns, which allow the use of Ag+ or enzymes would be very helpful. The benefit of analysing triglycerides this way was questioned.

A substantial part of the discussion focused on the relative merits of using fatty acid composition of different sampling sites (plasma, adipose tissue, red cell, platelet). It was agreed that for long-term monitoring of linoleic acid intake adipose tissue may be the best in view of integrated exposure, cost, well-validated, simplicity of analysis, though several queried whether compliance in studies in mediterranean countries would not be low when this procedure would be used. There was scepticism about the value of adipose tissue to monitor n-3 fatty acid intake. It was also agreed that for short-term dietary assessment, other fractions might be better. Some suggest phospholipids, erythrocytes or platelets particularly when n-3 diets are studied.

Concern is that stability of samples may differ, but in the hands of experts these oxidation problems can be overcome for all fractions.

The use of fatty acid composition as a biomarker to check on compliance in intervention studies was briefly discussed. In one study specific triglyceride species might be indicative of a vegetarian diet. It is worth mentioning that there is no marker for total fat intake or even for monoenoic or saturated fat intake at all. The use of a harmless marker (say ^{13}C-labelled fatty acids was mentioned) was suggested and this might have the additional advantage to give information on total fat consumption (by isotope dilution).

The possibility of using a biomarker for lipid peroxidation was mentioned, but although recognised as an important issue, it could not be discussed as few felt competent in this area.

The group felt that adipose linoleate as a marker of dietary intake is now widely recognised and this is perhaps the main highlight in this area. New techniques (NMR, new chromatographic methods) are being looked at and the initial results are exciting. The food composition data is a problem area, partly because of changing food availability (convenience foods) and food patterns, but also because of lack of information from the industry and lack or delay in updating of existing data. The use of fatty acid analysis of duplicate portions is perhaps more reliable, but is not practical for large surveys.

Several trials, both cross-sectional, retrospective and longitudinal are ongoing or are planned using adipose linoleate as a valid marker of dietary intake of this fatty acid.

Plasma fatty acid pattern as a biological marker for dietary intake of long chain n-3 fatty acids*

C.A. DREVON[1], K. SOLVOLL[1], K. LUND-LARSEN[1], B. SANDSTAD[1], T. TANDE[2], I. BAKSAAS[2] and E. SØYLAND[2]

[1]Section for Dietary Research, Institute for Nutrition Research, University of Oslo, [2]Norsk Hydro Research Center, Porsgrunn, Norway

Previous data from subjects supplied with different dietary fatty acids suggested that long chain n-3 fatty acids in plasma might be a useful marker of similar dietary fatty acids (1,2). In a double-blind clinical trial, 92 subjects out of total 241 patients with psoriasis or atopic dermatitis, were included to evaluate dietary and plasma fatty acids before and after intervention on the dietary fatty acid pattern.

Evaluation of dietary fatty acids was performed by using a newly developed selfadministered questionnaire, aiming at dietary history. The subjects were then randomized into two different groups, receiving gelatin capsules each containing one gram of either corn oil or highly concentrated n-3 fatty acids (K85, Norsk Hydro, containing > 95% n-3 fatty acids, eicosapentaenoic acid (EPA; 20:5, n-3) and docosahexaenoic acid (DHA; 22:6, n-3) accounting for at least 85% of total fatty acid content) daily. The patients were kept on this regime for 4 months. A new evaluation of dietary intake of fatty acids was performed using the selfadministered, optimal mark reading questionnaire. Venous blood samples were obtained from the subjects before and after the supplement with oils was provided, and the fatty acid pattern of plasma phospholipids was analyzed by gas liquid chromatography.

Correlations between plasma fatty acid concentrations and the corresponding food fatty acids showed that there were highly significant relations for EPA and DHA only, among all the 92 subjects, as well as among the subgroups of patients with atopic dermatitis and psoriasis. The correlation coefficients were 0.79 ($p < 0.0001$) for EPA and 0.42 ($p < 0.0001$) for DHA when all subjects were included. The highly significant correlations were also present after double-blind supplement of n-3 and n-6 fatty acids for 4 months. Even better correlations were obtained by considering the difference of plasma and food corresponding fatty acids before and after 4 months of supplement. In these situations correlations for Δ plasma fatty acids (after-before) to Δ corresponding dietary fatty acids (after-before were 0.81 ($p < 0.0001$) for EPA and 0.55 ($p < 0.0001$) for DHA, among all these 92 subjects. These data indicate that the plasma phospholipid fatty acid pattern can be used as a valuable biological marker for dietary intake of long chain n-3 fatty acids, at low as well as high intakes.

References

1 Bjørneboe et al. Br J Dermatol 1987;117:463-469.
2 Bjørneboe et al. Br J Dermatol 1988;118:77-83.

* Presented at plenary session

Triglyceride pattern of human sera as marker for vegetarian nutrition

H.U. MELCHERT and K. KEMPER

Institute for Social Medicine and Epidemiology of the Federal Health Office, Berlin, Germany

In the Berlin Vegetarian Study a method was developed that enables the separation and characterization of complex native triglycerides of serum samples. By combination of adsorption chromatography on $AgNO_3$ -impregnated silicagel mini-columns and RP-HPLC four characteristic triglyceride patterns can be obtained for each sample; reflecting the degree of saturation and chain length of fatty acids. The isocratic HPLC has been done with Hypersil ODS (5 μm) using propionitrile as eluent. The substances have been detected with a sensitive differential-refractometer. By semi-preparative work the different triglycerides were isolated and characterized by GLC of their fatty acid moieties.

A sample amount of 0.5–1.0 ml serum is sufficient to describe the triglyceride patterns. With this method the influence of a vegetarian diet on the composition of serum triglycerides has been examined in sera of vegetarians and non-vegetarians. Sera of vegetarians mostly contained triglycerides with polyunsaturated fatty acids (e.g. Dipalmitolinolein and Dioleolinolein) while non-vegetarian sera contained triglycerides with saturated fatty acids or with palmitoleic acid (e.g. Dipalmitoolein and Palmitodipalmitolein).

The method allows the observation of variations in serum triglycerides due to nutrition habits, due to sickness or due to medical treatment with lipid lowering agents affecting especially the triglyceride part of serum lipids.

Potential use of magnetic resonance spectroscopy to monitor compliance with taking fish oil supplements: a pilot study

P.C. DAGNELIE[1], J.D. BELL[1], H. PARKES[2] and T.A.B. SANDERS[3]

[1]NMR-Unit, Hammersmith Hospital; [2]Department of Chemistry, Birkbeck College; and [3]Department of Nutrition, Kings College, London, United Kingdom

Study questions

1. Does ^{31}P, ^{1}H and ^{13}C Nuclear Magnetic Resonance (NMR) Spectroscopy detect changes in plasma after short-term high-dose fish oil supplementation?
2. Can the changes detected by NMR be correlated with other biological indicators of Ω-3 fatty acids intake, such as plasma phospholipid composition or incorporation of Ω-3 fatty acids into red cell membranes?
3. Are changes of plasma NMR spectra correlated with changes of in-vivo NMR liver spectra?

Background

Ω-3 fatty acids from fish oil, especially eicosapentanoic acid (EPA) and docosahexanoic acid (DHA), have aroused increasing interest in the prevention and treatment of different diseases. Indicators of intake of Ω-3 fatty acids are therefore needed for measuring compliance in studies involving fish oil supplementation. The present pilot study was carried out to investigate whether in-vitro and/or in-vivo NMR Spectroscopy might be of use.

Subjects and methods

Five healthy male volunteers (30–45 years of age) on a usual low-fish diet (max. 1 meal with fish per week) were examined before (Day 0) and after (Days 3 and 7) taking a fish oil supplement providing approximately 10 g of EPA and 6.7 g of DHA. From one week before and throughout the study, all volunteers continued their usual diet but without any fish. Intravenous lithium heparin blood samples were obtained after fasting overnight (no food or caloric drinks for 12 hours). Plasma was stored at -20°C until analysis.

In-vitro ^{1}H NMR spectra were obtained on a 11.5 T magnet. Twodimensional ^{31}P chemical shift images of the liver were obtained on a 1.6 Picker whole body magnet using a saddle-shaped transmitter coil and a 15 cm surface receiver coil, using repetition times of 0.5, 1, and 5 s.

Results and discussion

All NMR spectra of plasma showed consistent changes that could be directly attributed to the intake of fish oil. In-vivo MR spectra revealed an increase in phosphodiester to ATP ratios. The time course of the NMR changes was directly related to the changes in plasma and red cell lipid composition measured by conventional methods.

Effect of the short-term day-to-day variability of serum lipids on the accuracy of CHD-risk assignment

C. SCACCINI[1], M. MARCELLI[2] and A. D'AMICIS[1]

[1]Human Nutrition Unit, National Institute of Nutrition, Rome, Italy;
[2]Clinical Nutrition Unit, Ospedale S. Spirito, Rome, Italy

Lowering blood cholesterol is a goal proposed from International Consensus Conferences to prevent heart diseases. Dietary and pharmacological interventions are also proposed for subjects classified at moderate- and high-risk serum cholesterol levels. These recommendations raise a question about the constancy of blood cholesterol levels and the reliability with which an individual is classified at the various levels of risk. There are three major sources of uncertainty in the measurement of plasma cholesterol (and lipids): imprecision, inaccuracy (which can be controlled by improving laboratory standardization and introducing calibrators and quality control procedures) and intra-individual biological and physiological variation.

The cause of this intra-individual variation is unknown. Some data show that the serum cholesterol level is far from constant even under metabolic ward conditions, but only few data refer to the elderly people. This study examines the impact of short-term intra-individual biologic variation of total cholesterol (TC), high-density lipoprotein cholesterol (HDL-C) and triglycerides (TG) on the CHD risk assignment in subjects belonging to different classes of age.

Up to date, fasting lipid values were measured on 25 healthy volunteers, (12 subjects under 40 and 13 over 60). Subjects were instructed to follow their typical diet following a 12-hour fast. Blood samples for lipid measurements were drawn on four mornings during 10 days. The proportion of biological variation was calculated according to the formula:

$$(\text{biological CV})^2 = (\text{total intra-individual CV})^2 - (\text{analytical CV})^2$$

Sensible day-to-day biological variation of TC (5%), HDL-C (5%) and TG (17%) was found. The biological variation shows the tendency to be lower in the older group than in the younger one. The difference reaches statistical significance in the case of the TG only (5%, by 2-factor ANOVA). By using $D_o = 1.96 * CV_{biol}/\sqrt{n}$, for the whole group it is possible to calculate that a single measure produces a percentage deviation from the "true" value (i.e. the mean of 4 measures) of 10% for TC (± 25 mg/dl) and for HDL-C (± 5 mg/dl), and of 34% for TG (39 mg/dl), at 95% probability. Using the mean of three measures, this deviation falls to 6% for TC and HDL-C and remains high for TG (± 20%). Due to the lower CV_{biol} in the older people, in this group the same level of accuracy is achieved with 2 measures only.

These results confirm that particular attention have to be paid to the day-to-day intra-individual variation to avoid the risk of misclassification. Furthermore, our findings seem to indicate that multiple measurements (>3 are particularly important to correctly classify the young group of subjects.

The correct classification of subjects should be considered fundamental to undertake any dietetic or pharmacological intervention for lowering blood-cholesterol.

Variability in cholesterol and fatty acids intake in the south of Spain. Something to consider when a biomarkers study is planned

J. GÓMEZ-ARACENA, F. RIUS DÍAZ, E. GÓMEZ GRACIA, A. PINEDO SANCHEZ and J. FERNÁNDEZ-CREHUET NAVAJAS

Departamento de Medicina Preventiva y Social, Facultad de Medicina, Málaga, Spain

Even when the influence of food intake on cholesterol and fatty acids as biomarkers, has been discussed, it is useful to know how this intake could change every day. This paper analyses their daily and seasonal variation. Using the 48-hour recall in two occasions in summer and winter (8 days in total), a dietary survey in 80 families, including 285 persons in a district of Málaga has been performed.

Applying the Friedman Test, significant differences were found during summer time in daily intake of total lipids, monounsaturated fatty acid, unsaturated fatty acid and oleic acid. While in winter there was not any variation.

Seasonal differences were also studied, using the t-Student test. It was found that the intake of PUFA, unsaturated fatty acid and linoleic acid was higher during summer.

It is important to remark that no seasonal or daily variation was found in the intake of cholesterol.

The main source of fatty acids was oil, specially olive oil and eggs contributed with more than 50% of cholesterol.

Questionnaire and tissue measures of dietary fat intake in Jerusalem

J.D. KARK, E.M. BERRY, Y. FRIEDLANDER and N.A. KAUFMANN

Hadassah University Hospital and Hebrew University-Hadassah; Faculty of Medicine, Israel

The Israeli diet is characterized by an increasing total fat intake over the past 25 years from an estimated 28% of total calories to 36% recently, and by a continuing high ratio of polyunsaturated to saturated (P:S) fatty acids. Total and cardiovascular mortality have reduced markedly over the past 2 decades. Our objective was to study the interrelationship of tissue and dietary measures of fatty acid composition. An age stratified random sample of the Jewish population of Jerusalem aged 25 to 64 was selected as a control group for a study of acute myocardial infarction; 817 men and women participated. Fatty acid composition of the diet was obtained by a semiquantitative food frequency questionnaire (82% response rate). The fatty acid composition of red blood cell membrane total phospholipids and subcutaneous adipose tissue aspirated from the buttock were measured in 570 and 558 people respectively (77% and 75% response). The proportion of SFA was 10.5% –10.9% of total calories with a P:S ratio of 0.8 to 0.9. About 30% of the population reported polyunsaturated fat intake of more than 10% of total calories. The proportion of linoleic acid in adipose tissue exceeded 25% (P:S ratio of 1.1), a high value in comparison with other countries. Associations between the different measures of fat composition are considered.

Polyunsaturated fatty acids in adipose tissue in 38-year old European men in relation to serum lipids, smoking habits, and fat distribution

J.C. SEIDELL[1], M. CIGOLINI[2], J. DESLYPERE[3], J. CHARZEWSKA[4], and B. ELLSINGER[5].

[1]Department of Human Nutrition, Agricultural University, Wageningen, The Netherlands; [2]Institute of Clinical Medicine, University of Verona, Italy; [3]Department of Endocrinology, University of Gent, Belgium; [4]National Institute of Food and Nutrition, Warsaw, Poland; [5]Department of Medicine I, University of Gothenburg, Sweden

Fat biopsies were taken from 327 38-year old men from 5 different European communities. Linoleic acid content varied widely ($F=110.6$, $p < 0.0001$) and was lowest in men from Poland (8.6%) and highest in men from Belgium (16.7%). Adipose tissue content of alpha-linolenic acid was subject to less variation ($F=13.9$, $p < 0.001$) and was lowest in men from Italy (0.52%) and highest in Sweden (0.89%). Correlations between linoleic acid and alpha-linolenic acid and serum lipids differed between the centers but in analysis combining information from all centers linoleic acid was negatively correlated to ldl-cholesterol (r-0.15, $p < 0.01$) and total cholesterol ($r=-0.17$, $p<0.01$). Alpha-linolenic acid was negatively correlated to serum triglycerides only ($r=-0.14$ $p < 0.05$). In analysis of covariance these associations remained after adjustment for smoking habits, body mass index, and waist/hip ratio. Together these variables could account for between 10.4% (ldl-cholesterol) and 26.2% (triglycerides) of the variation in serum lipids but failed to diminish the significant differences in hdl-cholesterol and triglycerides that were observed between the different populations.

We conclude that long-term biomarkers of fatty acid intake are related to short-term indicators of lipid metabolism.

The fatty acid composition of plasma fatty acids after diets high in rapeseed oil or sunflower oil

I. AHOLA[1], A. ARO[1], M JAUHIAINEN[1], L.M. VALSTA[2], and M. MUTANEN[2]

[1]National Public Health Institute, Helsinki and [2]Dept. of Nutrition, University of Helsinki, Finland

In a randomized crossover study 30 women and 29 men consumed diets high in rapeseed oil (RO) or sunflower oil (SO) for 3.5 weeks after a preceding 2-week baseline diet (BAS) high in saturated fat (SAFA). Intakes of total fat, cholesterol, and fish were similar during the diets.

diet	SAFA	MUFA	n-6 PUFA	n-3 PUFA (en%)
BAS	19	11	3.7	
RO	12	16	5.6	2.0
SO	13	10	13	

The fatty acid composition of serum phospholipids (PL), cholesterol esters (CE) and triglycerides (TG) were determined by gas chromatography as methyl esters. The RO diet increased the proportion of oleic acid in PL from 12% to 13% and the SO diet the proportion of linoleic acid from 25 to 31% compared to BAS diet. The α-linolenic acid in RO diet increased the relative amount of this fatty acid three-fold in TG compared to BAS. Eicosapentaenoic acid (EPA) in PL increased less: When RO diet followed the BAS diet the proportion of EPA increased from 1.0% to 1.5% ($p < 0.01$). In the other group on SO diet the competition between n-6 and n-3 fatty acids decreased the proportion of EPA from 1.4% to 0.6% ($p < 0.01$) compared to the BAS situation. The findings suggest that in man α-linolenic acid from rapeseed oil is metabolized to EPA to a very limited extent.

11

Workshop III: Selenium

Biomarkers of selenium: workshop report
PIETER van 't VEER and GEORG ALFTHAN

Deposition of selenium in toenails is dependent on the form of dietary selenium
G. ALFTHAN et al.

Can serum selenium be used as an indicator of selenium intake?
H.M. MELTZER et al.

Glutathione peroxidase activity as an indicator of the human selenium status
A. ARO et al.

Glutathione peroxidase activity as a biomarker of the selenium status of man
A. van FAASSEN et al.

Is human hair a suitable indicator for body selenium status?
J.J.M. de GOEIJ et al.

Intra- and interindividual variance of toenail concentrations of selenium, calcium, zinc, magnesium, sodium, and copper
H. BOEING et al.

Predictors of toenail selenium in men and women
P.A. van den BRANDT et al.

Biomarkers of dietary exposure. Ed. F. J. Kok & P. van 't Veer.

Biomarkers of selenium: workshop report

PIETER van 't VEER[1] and GEORG ALFTHAN[2]

[1]Epidemiology Section, TNO Toxicology and Nutrition Institute, Zeist, Netherlands; [2]National Public Health Institute, Helsinki, Finland

The health relevance of selenium is obvious from various phenomena, among others its recognition as an essential trace element incorporated in the enzyme glutathione peroxidase (GSH-Px), the preventive effect of selenium in Keshan disease, and the inverse association between selenium and both cardiovascular as well as malignant disease. Because the fluctuating selenium content of food products prohibits reliable assessment of selenium intake, the need for biomarkers of selenium intake has been recognized by nutritional epidemiologists for a long time. Both the potential health relevance of selenium, as well as the difficulties in reliable assessment of individual selenium intake have contributed to substantial research on biomarkers of selenium during the past decade.

Biomarkers of selenium intake can be classified into GSH-Px-activity and selenium-concentrations in various tissues (media). Selection of the optimal biomarker in a given research setting depends on the level of selenium intake within the population and the time integrating properties of the biological medium. Clarity has emerged on the properties of these biomarkers of selenium intake.

Activity of GSH-Px is sensitive to dietary intake, but plateaus in plasma at an intake of about 50 μg/day, in erythrocytes at 60–80 μg/day and in platelets at some level above 120 μg/day. In selenium supplementation studies, platelet activity and plasma values respond within several days, but erythrocytes seem to have more time-integrating properties. Because of the plateau, a high response to supplementation is observed among populations with low selenium status (Figure 1). Although GSH-Px assessment as such is relatively simple, a reference for standardization of GSH-Px activity is not available. Therefore, activities assessed by different labs or from different time periods within the same lab cannot be compared and the level of selenium intake needs to be accounted for.

Selenium concentrations in urine, plasma, erythrocytes, and hair or toenails have increasing time-integrating properties ranging from one day, several days to one week, several months and several months to half a year respectively. Urinary selenium is considered an adequate biomarker of individual selenium intake, provided repeated urine-collections and balanced intake and output.

For applications in etiologic research in nutritional epidemiology, feasibility and time-integrating properties of biomarkers are of great importance, the latter especially in retrospective studies. From this viewpoint, hair and (toe)nails have great potential as biomarkers. However, since hair is more prone to contamination, nails appear to be more suited. Nevertheless, data

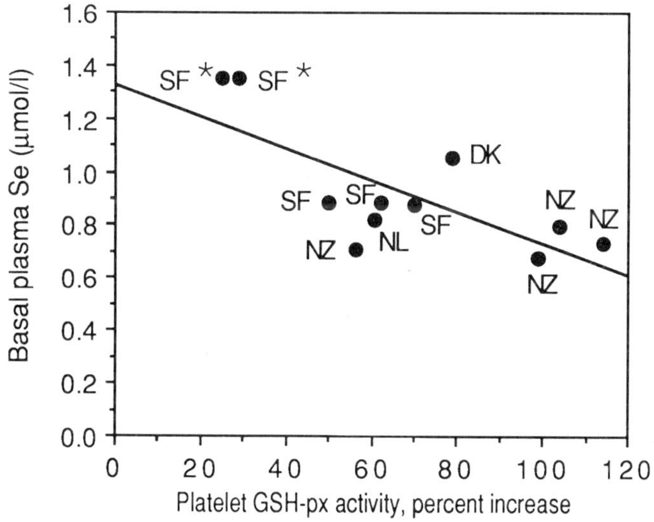

FIGURE 1. Percent increase of platelet GSH-Px activity at plateau during selenium supplementation in relation to basal plasma selenium concentration. SF*=Finland during selenium fertilization, SF=Finland before selenium fertilization, DK=Denmark, NL=Netherlands, NZ=New Zealand (adapted from Alfthan et al. Am J Clin Nutr 1991;53:120–125).

on selenium levels in hair show significant correlation with liver selenium values for Asians, though less so for Europeans. Hair selenium may be a useful indicator in countries with a large heterogeneity, e.g. in Asia, while less so in Europe (Figure 2; results from the IAEA coordinated research programme on the significance of hair mineral analysis as means for assessing internal body burdens of environmental pollutants). Furthermore, liver selenium levels are in their turn correlated with selenium levels in various other tissues, suggesting that selenium stores are distributed over the body, rather than concentrated in a particular tissue. These results are encouraging for (toe)nails as biomarker for selenium status.

In order to take full advantage of toenails as biomarker of selenium status, attention should be given to within-study standardization and adequate description of nail collection (big toes only, or all toes), and sample preparation (debris, nail polish) and analytical aspects (water content, particle size). External reference materials are available and should be used to enhance between-laboratory and international comparisons. These materials are useful independent of the analytical methods, e.g. Atomic Absorption Spectrometry (AAS) or Instrumental Neutron Activation Analysis (INAA).

Although much has become clear the past decade on biomarkers of selenium intake, their relative sensitivity to dietary intake remains to be determined, as well as their sensitivity to other lifestyle factors and the potential role in disease etiology.

First, the sensitivity of these different biomarkers to dietary intake is largely based on cross-sectional studies and needs further elaboration in experimental

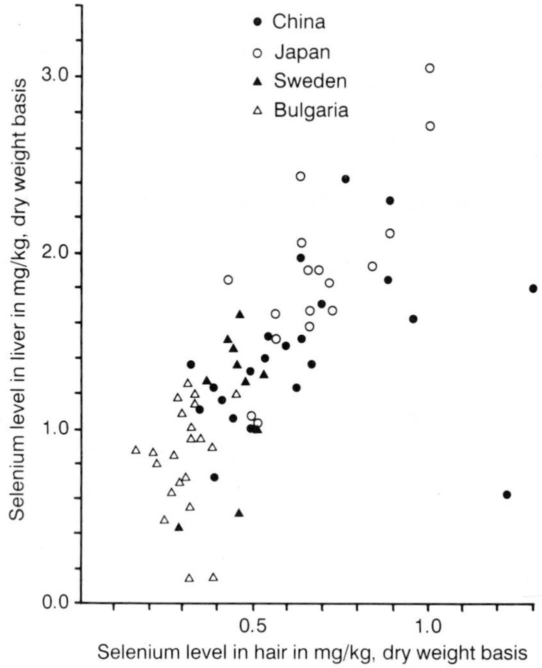

FIGURE 2. Hair selenium versus liver selenium for residents from China, Japan, Bulgaria and Sweden. Data from both Asian countries show a strong and significant correlation between liver selenium and hair selenium, viz. r=0.78 (n=17) and r=0.57 (n=24). For both European countries the degree of correlation is much weaker and not significant, viz. r=0.10 (n=21) and r=0.38 (n=11) respectively (IAEA results, see text and abstract by J.J.M. de Goeij et al).

research. Thus, uptake and distribution of inorganic (e.g., selenite, selenate) and organic forms of selenium (selenocysteïne and selenomethionine) or from major food sources (e.g. meat, fish and grain products) or supplements needs to be clarified, both regarding selenium concentrations and GSH-Px activity in biological media. In this respect, knowledge of selenium as related to cancer may be as incomplete as knowledge on fatty acids in relation to cardiovascular disease few decades ago.

Second, selenium-status seems to be lower in males, current smokers and subjects with high body weight. Thus, in validation studies selenium biomarkers may better reflect dietary intake when these factors are taken into account. In etiologic research, however, the biomarker as such may be relevant to disease occurrence, and removing part of its heterogeneity by adjustment for these covariates in multivariate analysis may reduce the association between the biomarker and outcome.

Regarding disease etiology, the essential role of selenium in GSH-Px and antioxidant properties of other selenium compounds suggest that an antioxidant function of selenium might be important. In this realm, further research needs to take into account other food constituents with antioxidant properties as well (e.g. α-tocopherol, β-carotene, ascorbic acid). It is interesting that biomarkers of several of these latter food-related antioxidants are also lowered in smoking subjects.

The search for other selenium-containing proteins is still in progress. At present, however, there are no indications that this will result in biomarkers of either internal or biologically effective dose. Furthermore, though lowered selenium levels have been used as "cancer markers" long ago, they are unlikely to emerge as useful biomarkers of disease progression or early outcome in epidemiologic research.

The hypothesis that selenium reduces cancer risk dates essentially from ecological research, followed by retrospective and nested case-control studies in low selenium areas as New Zealand and Finland, respectively. Although some of these studies tended to support the hypothesis, results have not been fully consistent with studies in intermediate or high selenium areas. Most prospective studies, however, did not permit powerful site-specific data-analysis and, therefore, are restricted to total cancer risk. Case-control studies have been directed at the most frequent malignancy among women in affluent societies, i.e. breast cancer, but the postulated inverse association could not be substantiated. For organs and tissues more directly affected by environmental exposures, such as the lungs (smoking) and gastrointestinal sites (diet), the role of selenium remains to be determined. Several studies that include selenium biomarkers are in progress.

Further improvement in nutritional epidemiologic studies on selenium could be obtained by considering more specific disease categories and the time aspect of disease occurrence. Thus, although the role of selenium in cardiovascular disease was not extensively discussed in the workshop, one should clearly distinguish the role of selenium during the course of atherogenesis, the acute event of thrombogenesis and the oxidant stress following myocardial infarction. In cancer etiology, it may be fruitful to study disease precursors like proliferative disease and atypical hyperplasia breast cancer. For colon cancer, polyps may serve as an intermediate endpoint or as starting point for intervention studies. For lung cancer, indicators of effective dose to oxidant stress among smokers (SCEs, micronuclei, adducts) may be used as markers of a diminished biologically effective dose due to favorable selenium status.

Thus, much quantitative information has become available on the characteristics of biomarkers of total selenium intake. Because a reliable assessment of selenium intake by dietary methodology is extremely difficult, these biomarkers are essential to study the health effects of this trace element. The public health relevance to populations with marginal or normal selenium intake has to be evaluated for both specific disease outcomes and disease precursors, as well as in combination with (biomarkers of) other antioxidant food constituents.

Deposition of selenium in toenails is dependent on the form of dietary selenium*

G. ALFTHAN, A. ARO, H. ARVILOMMI and J.K. HUTTUNEN

National Public Health Institute, Helsinki, Finland

Toenails are becoming an increasingly attractive tissue for assessing the long-term dietary intake of selenium (Se). Sampling is noninvasive, samples are easy to store and they afford integrated data over several months. However, experiments with Se-deficient rats show that the dietary Se intake level and the chemical form of Se influence the deposition of Se in nails. We studied the deposition of Se with either Se-enriched yeast (mainly selenomethionine), selenite or selenate (200 μg Se/d) for 16 weeks in toenails in a placebo-controlled supplementation study in healthy men with a basal Se intake of 100 μg/d. Toenail clippings are acquired at baseline and 10 and 32 weeks after supplementation ceased. In separate in vitro experiments we also studied effects of washing procedures on the Se concentration of nails.

Toenail Se concentration (mean ± SD) increased ($P<0.01$) from 9.16 ± 0.92 to 11.2 ± 1.11 μmol/kg in the group receiving Se-yeast compared to placebo. The other chemical forms of Se were not deposited in toenails.

Of all samples 6.7% were excluded as outliers due to possible contamination by Se-containing shampoo. Treatment of nail clippings with diluted (0.1%) Se-shampoo (2.5% Se) resulted in a 40-fold increase in the Se concentration. This external Se could not be removed by extracting with any of 9 different reagents. The most successful reagent was acidic stannous/chloride, which removed 70% of the external Se.

Toenails reflect Se intake from diets rich in selenomethionine, such as grains but not from inorganic Se compounds.

* Presented at plenary session

Can serum selenium be used as an indicator of selenium intake

H.M. MELTZER[1] and K. BIBOW[2]

[1]Institute for Nutrition Research and [2]Department of Chemistry, University of Oslo, Oslo, Norway

Following many studies showing connections between health conditions and indicators of selenium status, serum selenium has been suggested as a biological marker of Se intake. There is generally a good correlation between serum Se and Se intake at low intakes, although important counterexamples are known. However, recent models of human Se metabolism (e.g. the selenite-exchangable-pool model proposed by Janghorbani and Young) suggest that the relation between intake and status is, generally, complicated. Studies conducted on relatively Se-replete populations (e.g. Norwegians: Average serum Se ca 120 µg/Lg seem to support this. They clearly demonstrate that serum Se, may *not* – in general – be used as an indicator of Se intake. Here are some findings from our group:

1. In two independent studies, the correlation between Se intake, found by analyzing duplicate portions, and serum Se, were r=0.32 (n=16) and r=0.29 (n=32), respectively.
2. A two-fold increase in dietary Se intake, in the form of fish, did note affect serum Se, and actually *lowered* platelet Se.
3. Se from Se-rich wheat consistently raised serum Se levels, in a dose-dependent manner.
4. Supplementation with 200 µg Se as pea-powder did not influence serum Se.
5. Supplementation with 200 µg Se as yeast Se raised serum Se significantly.

In conclusion, there may be a number of factors which influence the serum response to dietary Se intake. Moreover, these factors probably introduce systematic bias into attempts at estimating Se intake from serum values in relatively Se-replete populations.

Glutathione peroxidase activity as an indicator of the human selenium status

A. ARO, G. ALFTHAN, H. ARVILOMMI and J.K. HUTTUNEN

National Public Health Institute, Helsinki, Finland

Maximal activity of glutathione peroxidase (GSHPx) in various tissues has been used to estimate the selenium (Se) requirement of animals. In humans, maximal activity of GSHPx in plasma occurs at an Se intake of 50 µg/d and in red cells at an estimated intake of 60-80 µg/d. The daily intake required for maximal activity of the enzyme in platelets is not known. Two placebo-controlled Se supplementation studies with a time interval of six years were conducted in men, the first (A) at a basal Se intake of 55 µg/dF (200 mg Se/d for 11 weeks as Se-rich yeast, wheat or selenate) and the second (B) at 100 µg/d (200 µg Se/d for 16 weeks as Se-rich yeast, selenite or selenate) during the addition of Se to fertilizers. The corresponding mean plasma Se concentrations at baseline were 0.88 and 1.39 µmol/l. In study (A) all forms of Se induced maximal GSHPx activity in platelets after 4 weeks, the increase compared to placebo ranging form 50% to 70%. In study (B) selenite and selenate induced an increase of c. 30%, whereas Se-yeast did not significantly stimulate enzyme activity. Plasma and red cell GSHPx activities were not stimulated by any forms of Se in either study. Linear regression analysis of the present data and published data from studies of similar design (200–256 µg Se/d, 8-32 weeks) suggests that maximal platelets GSHPx activity occurs at a plasma Se concentration of 1.2–1.5 µmol/l. We conclude that in the assessment of the Se status using GSHPx as an indicator it is essential to estimate the level of dietary Se intake before choosing the tissue to be assayed for GSHPx activity.

Glutathione peroxidase activity as a biomarker of the selenium status of man

A. van FAASSEN[3], J. ENGELEN[2], H.E. FALKE[1] and R.J.J. HERMUS[1]

[1]TNO Toxicology and Nutrition Institute, Zeist, The Netherlands; [2]Department of Clinical Genetics, University of Limburg, Maastricht, The Netherlands; [3]PBI B.V., Maastricht, The Netherlands

Selenium (Se) status as measured by the serum concentration of Se has been associated negatively with the risk of gastrointestinal cancer in prospective studies in countries with intermediate Se-status. We studied the feasibility of the activity of the Se-dependent enzyme glutathione peroxidase (GSH-Px) in plasma as a biomarker requiring little biological material by:

1. developing a rapid and reproducible method of analysis requiring less than 0.1 ml plasma
2. analyzing the intra- to interindividual variability of the marker
3. correlating plasma GSH-Px activity in a cross-sectional study with:
   a) GSH-Px activity in red blood cells
   b) Se-concentration in serum,
   c) Se-intake from the diet.

Plasma is separated from red and white blood cells by centrifuging for 10 minutes at 1500 g in a simple desk centrifuge. Platelet poor plasma (ppp) is made by centrifuging blood for 30 minutes at 1500 g. The plasma GSH-Px activity is measured with the Cobas Bio centrifugal analyzer (Hoffman la Roche). This allows to analyze twenty-four samples in half an hour with an intra-run coefficient of variation of 3%.

The intra- to interindividual variability of the plasma GSH-Px activity, calculated from 4 samples separated by a week of 6 male volunteers between 20 and 40 yrs was 0.03, while it was 0.56 for GSH-Px activity in red blood cells.

The correlation of the plasma GSH-Px activity with those in red blood cells was 0.68 (Pearson coefficient of correlation, $p<0.05$, measured in 6 male volunteers between 20 to 40 years).

The ppp GSH-Px activity was significantly associated with the Se-concentration in serum of 42 Dutch men and women (Spearman coefficient of correlation = 0.35, $p<0.05$) and with the intake of Se from the diet (Pearson coefficient of correlation = 0.32, $p<0.05$; mean ± standard deviation of Se-intake = 60 ± 16 µg/day). In literature it is shown that the activity of GSH-Px in platelets and in ppp respond to changes in Se-intake.

In conclusion the plasma GSH-Px activity is preferred as a biomarker for the Se-status, because:

a) it can be measured quickly and reproducible in a small amount of biological material
b) it has a low intra- to interindividual variation
c) it correlates significantly with and responds to changes in the Se-intake.

Is human hair a suitable indicator for body selenium status?

J.J.M. de GOEIJ, M. BLAAUW and C. ZEGERS

Interfaculty Reactor Institute, Delft University of Technology, Delft, The Netherlands

In the frame of an IAEA-coordinated research programme on the significance of hair mineral analysis as a means for assessing internal body burdens of environmental pollutants, data have been collected on selenium in hair and a few tissues from autopsied males. The data were assessed for the analytical quality using detection limits and data for selenium levels in certified reference materials and "blind" samples. The analytical quality of the data from four countries was sufficient for further data handling. Selenium levels in hair tend to be higher in the Far East (Japan and China) than in Europe (Sweden and Bulgaria), viz 0.65 ± 0.24 mg/kg and 0.67 ± 0.16 mg/kg versus 0.44 ± 0.06 mg/kg and 0.31 ± 0.06 mg/kg. Smoking and obesity were associated with a 10–15% lower hair selenium level. Hair colour, degree of urbanization, age, and cause of death did not exhibit an influence on hair selenium levels.

For the Asian samples a strong and significant correlation between hair selenium and liver selenium was found. In the European samples this correlation was much weaker and not significant. The pooled data show that above a hair selenium level of ca 0.4 mg/kg selenium levels in hair are well correlated with those in liver, while below this value hair selenium levels are rather independent of liver selenium levels. This makes hair not a useful indicator for body selenium status in Europeans.

Selenium levels in kidney, liver, spleen and heart were significantly correlated, indicating that for selenium no particular tissue (for instance the liver) is involved in selenium storage, but that selenium stores are distributed over the body.

Intra- and interindividual variance of toenail concentrations of selenium, calcium, zinc, magnesium, sodium, and copper

H. BOEING, N. BENSALEH and H. WESCH

Institute of Epidemiology and Biometry, German Cancer Research Center, Heidelberg, Germany

Toenail analysis is proposed to serve as biochemical indicator for dietary intake of minerals or trace elements. This study evaluated for which of the 6 elements being tested sufficient inter-individual variation compared to intra-individual variation existed in order to refer to individual exposure in a single toenail sample.

Material and methods

35 males and females of all age groups provided in a consequentive way toenail clippings in the range of 2 to 7 times, 26 of them 3 or 4 samples. These toenail clippings were washed and solved in H_2O_2 and HNO_3. Selenium and zinc were determined by neutron activation and calcium, magnesium, sodium and copper by atomic absorption spectroscopy.

Results

The mean concentration of all 116 samples from the 35 individuals, weighted by the reciprocal of the number of samples per individual, was for selenium 0.44 μg/g toenail clipping, zinc 119 μg/g, calcium 848 μg/g, magnesium 83.9 μg/g, sodium 385 μg/g, and copper 6.9 μg/g. The concentration of calcium, sodium, and copper were slightly higher among males. The percentages of inter- and intra-individual variance and the coefficients of variation (CV) for the mean values of the individuals were as indicated in table 1.

TABLE 1. Intra- and inter-individual variance of minerals or trace elements in toenails

	selenium	zinc	calcium	magnesium	sodium	copper
intra-individual (per cent)	50	19	22	52	64	90
inter-individual (per cent)	50	81	78	48	36	10
CV	14	29	66	55	82	39

Discussion

The approach of measuring mineral or trace element intake, throughout toenail concentration seems most promising for calcium because of stable estimates among individuals in different time periods and also of high variation between individuals, followed by zinc which did show less variation. Selenium and magnesium showed a much higher intra-individual variability. For these elements, a single toenail clipping is associated with increased exposure misclassification. The analysis of copper or sodium in a single toenail sample allows no particular reference to the individual situation. The study did not test whether toenail concentrations of mineral and trace elements in individuals reflect their dietary intake of the set elements.

Predictors of toenail selenium in men and women

P.A. van den BRANDT[1], R.A. GOLDBOHM[2], P. van 'T VEER[2], P. BODE[3], R.J.J. HERMUS[2] and F STURMANS[1]

[1]Department of Epidemiology, University of Limburg, Maastricht, The Netherlands; [2]TNO Toxicology and Nutrition Institute, Zeist, The Netherlands; [3]Interfaculty Reactor Institute, Delft University of Technology, Delft, The Netherlands

Within a prospective cohort study (n=120, 852) on diet and cancer among men and women aged 55–69 years, toenail clippings were collected at baseline as a biomarker for long-term selenium status. The association between toenail selenium and gender, age and smoking status was investigated among a random subset of the cohort (558 men, 570 women). Subjects with prevalent cancer have been excluded from this subset. The selenium content of the toenail specimens was determined by instrumental neutron activation analysis. The mean toenail selenium level among all subjects was 0.56 ppm (standard deviation, SD: 0.11 ppm). Men were found to have significantly lower mean toenail selenium levels than women (mean ± SD: 0.55 ± 0.10 versus 0.58 ± 0.10 ppm, respectively; $p < 0.001$). Age was not related to toenail selenium concentration in the studied 15-year age range. Current smokers showed significantly lower mean toenail selenium levels than never smokers (mean ± SD: 0.53 ± 0.10 versus 0.58 ± 0.11 ppm, respectively; $p < 0.001$), with ex-smokers showing intermediate values (mean ± SD: 0.57 ± 0.10 ppm). Gender and smoking status persisted as independent predictors of toenail selenium concentration in multiple regression analysis.

This study is supported by the European Commission, the Dutch Cancer Society and the Dutch Ministry of Welfare, Public Health and Cultural Affairs.

12

Workshop IV: Antioxidants and minor food constituents

Biomarkers of dietary exposure. Ed. F. J. Kok & P. van 't Veer.

Relationships among diet, urinary nitrogen excretion and growth of the elementary school children in urban and rural areas of Korea
H.Y. PAIK

The use of individual biomarkers for improving and validating household salt consumption data
C. LECLERCQ

Development of biomarkers and elucidation of pathogenesis – the example of konzo, a newly identified nutritional myelopathy
H. RÖSLING

Biomarkers of antioxidants and minor food constituents: workshop report

FRED GEY and SEAN J. STRAIN

University of Bern, Bern, Switzerland; University of Ulster, Coleraine, Northern Ireland, United Kingdom

The formal presentations at this workshop consisted of a heterogenous collection of: two papers on associations between dietary and serum antioxidants; three papers on iron status measurements including their relationship to dietary iron intake; one paper on relationships between dietary protein and growth of children; one paper on the use of biomarkers for improving and validating household salt consumption data; and one paper on the development of blood cyanide level as a good biomarker of the combined effect of high cyanide and low sulphur intakes in the elucidation of the pathogenesis of a newly identified nutritional myelopathy.

Important considerations arising out of the papers on antioxidants were firstly that sex differences in serum retinol and β-carotene and smoking effects on serum β-carotene could still be detected even after up to 15 years storage of serum at –20°C (which is known to destroy a major fraction of antioxidants). Jarvinen et al. also found correlations between dietary and serum β-carotene in non-smoking men. Thamm et al. showed correlations of blood levels in the same individuals taken at two different times of year (Spring and Autumn) for serum vitamin C, vitamin E, carotenoids and vitamin A. This suggests that a single blood sample is suitable to characterize the gross status of essential antioxidants. The authors also demonstrated a moderate correlation between dietary and serum vitamin C when the latter was below the renal threshold.

Highlights from the iron papers included the following. Haraldsdóttir et al. obtained similar prevalences of iron deficiency for Danish women using serum ferritin cut-off points and probability calculations from dietary data. However, it remains to be elucidated whether this is a generalizable phenomenon. Data were presented by Duggan et al. to indicate that the zinc protoporphyrin test was a promising supplementary test for children at risk of iron deficiency and a correlation was found by Fricker et al. between iron status and obesity in pre-menopausal women.

The remaining papers in the workshop also provided some interesting data. A presentation by Paik, demonstrated correlations between growth parameters and protein, particularly animal protein in children in urban and rural areas of Korea. The disappearance of household salt could, after appropriate adjustments, be used for salt consumption of families as demonstrated by Leclerq et al. Finally Rosling presented evidence that blood cyanide was a good biomarker of the exposure to cassava roots which contain cytogenic glycosides. Further, the combined effect of high levels of blood cyanide and low sulphur intakes appeared to be the aetiological factor in the acute onset of a progressive aspastic paraparesis, known as Konzo in parts of Africa.

From the general discussion following the formal presentations in this workshop it was concluded that future research should: (a) improve and standardize storage conditions of antioxidants biomarkers; (b) explore further the adjustment for concurrent serum lipids with respect to lipid soluble antioxidants; (c) update food tables with respect to the micronutrients and to encourage, if possible, the food industry to label the actual antioxidant content; (d) make greater effort to link biomarkers, functional characteristics and disease processes related to specific nutrients. In general, most biomarkers, in spite of specific limitations, appear to be more informative for some nutrients than dietary assessments in applications to aetiological studies, nutritional monitoring studies and randomized trials.

Antioxidants in human serum: their relationship with constituents of the diet*

J. JÄRVISALO, J. MARNIEMI, A. LEINO, L. REHNBERG, M. AHOTUPA, P. PUUKKA, M. RASTAS and A. SEPPÄNEN

The Rehabilitation Research Centre of the Social Insurance Institute, Turku, Finland

In principle, there are two means to assess human antioxidant function: either one may expose a tissue specimen to an oxidative stress and follow the development of the oxidative damage. Or one may analyze a set of antioxidants, including various antioxidant vitamins and trace elements and enzymes, peroxidizable fatty acids and markers of the oxidative damage, such as lipid peroxides in the specimens.

Our approach in studies related to human antioxidant function has been to assess the role of antioxidants in secondary prevention of common chronic diseases. We have also tried to analyze the sources of variation of various components of the antioxidant function in human serum. Due to that we have performed several substudies which have included the use of a standardized diet, α-tocopherol/β-carotene intervention and a short term exposure to physical exercise. We have also assessed the need for fasting in standardizing the specimen collection for the measurements. The various components of the antioxidant function measured have included serum lipids, in some substudies also their individual fatty acids and vitamins A, C and E, β-carotene, Cu, Zn and Se. The measures for serum lipid peroxides used have been the diene conjugates and TBA-reactive material in serum. In the various substudies performed the food intake has been assessed with a food record or with an interview. The quantities of the various nutrients have been calculated with the aid of a computer based nutrient calculation programme (NUTRICA). Information on self-medication with drugs containing vitamins or trace elements has also been obtained. In a substudy in which the participants (n = 12) were on their normal diet while keeping a food record with household measures for two weeks, serum cholesterol levels did not show any correlation with the intake of cholesterol during the preceeding 3 days but was negatively correlated with P/S of the food during these days. Serum triglycerides were positively correlated with the fat intake. The serum levels of β-carotene showed a positive correlation with its intake but no correlation was seen between the levels of α-tocopherol, ascorbate, copper or zinc in serum and their intake during these days. Neither did the levels of diene conjugates or TBA-reactive material in serum correlate with the intake of polyunsaturated fatty acids.

Our information seems to indicate that the short-term intake of antioxidants cannot predict their levels in serum. It may be that any query based individual means of obtaining information on current or typical food intake may prove poor in this respect. Additionally, as observed in various intervention studies, there is a great individual serum level variation in response to antioxidant drugs, suggesting that the levels of these compounds in serum are suitable for assessing the antioxidant function in large scale epidemiological studies only.

*Presented at plenary session

Water-soluble vitamin biomarkers as indicators of "usual" vitamin intake*

M.J. KRETSCH, A.K.H. FONG and H.E. SAUBERLICH

USDA/ARS, Western Human Nutrition Research Center, San Francisco, CA, and Department of Nutritional Sciences, University of Alabama, Birmingham AL, USA

Biomarkers of thiamin, riboflavin, folate, vitamin B-6, and vitamin C were studied to determine their effectiveness in validating the "usual" vitamin intakes of individuals. Twenty-one, nonsmoking, healthy adults (9 women, 12 men) between 21–35 years of age were confined to a metabolic unit for 52 days. Physical activity was maintained at a constant level throughout the study for each subject, but was variable among subjects. The subjects were provided a diverse, 8-day rotating menu from which they were allowed free choice in deciding what and how much to eat. Dietary intake was precisely weighed and recorded for 32 days by trained dietary staff, and the mean vitamin intake for each individual calculated from food composition tables. Fasting blood samples (0830h) were drawn throughout the study at 8-day intervals, and the various biomarkers determined: erythrocyte transketolase activity coefficient (ETK-AC) for thiamin, erythrocyte glutathione reductase activity coefficient (EGR-AC) for riboflavin, erythrocyte aspartate transaminase activity coefficient (EAST-AC) for vitamin B-6, plasma and RBC folate, and plasma ascorbate. Using six blood samples per subject, within- to between-person variance ratios (W:B) for each biomarker were calculated for the males and females separately. W:B ratios were < 1.0 for EGR-AC, EAST-AC, and plasma ascorbate for both males and females, for plasma and RBC folacin for the males, and for ETK-AC for the females. Based on the W:B ratios and using the equation of Liu et al.[1], it was found that 3–4 blood samples per person were required for the majority of indicators in order to limit the dietary/biomarker correlation coefficient attenuation to $\leq 10\%$. Pearson correlation coefficients between the mean biomarker level (4 blood samples/subject) and the concurrent, mean dietary intake (mean of 32 days/subject) yielded significant correlations between vitamin C intake and plasma ascorbate for the male and female groups (+0.61 and +0.68, $p < 0.05$, respectively) and between vitamin B-6 intake and EAST-AC for the male group (–0.56, $p < 0.05$). These correlation coefficients apply to vitamin C intakes ranging between 42–356 mg/d and 97–302 mg/d for the males and females, respectively; and vitamin B-6 intakes ranging between 0.87–2.41 mg/d for the males. Plasma ascorbate and EAST-AC exhibit good potential as dietary validation tools for an individual's longterm vitamin C and B-6 intake but require further study under field conditions.

References

1 Liu K et al. J Chron Dis 1978;31:399

* Presented at plenary session

Dietary associations of serum β-carotene and serum retinol

R. JÄRVINEN[1] P. KNEKT[2], R.K. AARAN[3] and R. SEPPÄNEN[2]

[1]Department of Nutrition, University of Kuopio, Finland; [2]Research Institute for Social Security, Social Insurance Institution, Helsinki, Finland; [3]Department of Biomedical Sciences, University of Tampere, Finland

The associations of serum β-carotene and serum retinol concentrations with dietary data were studied among 341 adult men and women who represented serum controls of the cancer incidence follow-up study of the Finnish Mobile Clinic Health Survey. Field study was performed during 1968–1973. Serum samples were kept deepfrozen at –20°C until analyzed in 1984. The intakes of major dietary carotenoids, retinoids and total vitamin A were calculated from dietary history interviews covering the habitual diet of subjects over one-year period.

Serum β-carotene levels were higher in women (mean 125 μg/l) than in men (mean 86 μg/l), whereas serum retinol values were higher for men (mean 673 μg/l) than for women (mean 616 mg/l). Serum β-carotene and dietary β-carotene adjusted for important confouding factors were positively correlated in women ($r=0.38$, $p < 0.001$). Since the intakes of different dietary carotenoids were highly correlated, positive associations between these and serum β-carotene were also seen. Men who were current smokers had significantly lower serum β-carotene levels compared to nonsmokers, furthermore there was a significant interaction between smoking and dietary β-carotene in predicting serum β-carotene level. Positive association between serum and dietary β-carotene was found in nonsmoker-men, but not in current smokers. A tendency for association between serum β-carotene and dietary total vitamin A was seen in women, but not in men, which apparently was due to the greater contribution of carotenoids to the total vitamin A intake in women. Serum retinol levels were not significantly related to the intake of retinoids, carotenoids or total vitamin A.

This study supports earlier findings that smoking modifies the association between dietary β-carotene and serum β-carotene, and shows that even after 10 to 15 years of storage serum β-carotene can be an acceptable biochemical marker for dietary β-carotene.

The behaviour of selected biomarkers of naturally occurring antioxidants

M. THAMM, J. REHM and L. KOHLMEIER

Federal Health Office, WHO Collaborating Centre for Nutritional Epidemiology, Berlin, Germany

Biomarkers of dietary intake are the method of choice when they can provide reliable and valid information on the relative levels of the nutrients of interest, or serve as a latent variable for dietary intake. Because of the current interest in antioxidants, we examined the relationships of serum levels of vitamin A, β-carotene, ascorbic acid and tocopherol in serum of elderly and younger subjects, from which 7 day dietary records and 24 hour recall information was available for the period of time of the phlebotomy. Most subjects were examined at two times, in spring and in fall.

In the following, the results for the older group (age 65–74) will be presented. The pooled mean energy consumption stayed very much the same (55508 kJ/week in spring, and 57127 kJ/week in fall).

The results show a correlation (Pearson) of blood levels in the same individual at two different times of year of 0.67 for vitamin A, 0.76 for carotenoid, 0.70 for vitamin E, and 0.42 for vitamin C. Dietary intakes are expectedly less stable. Comparing the nutrient intake per week, according to a 7-day written dietary protocol, the correlation between spring and fall is lower than one would expect from the blood levels: 0.20 for vitamin A, 0.34 for vitamin E, and 0.41 for vitamin C. The levels of misclassification with the biomarkers, as compared with the dietary intake measurements were such that 14% suffered a more than two quintile shift in relationship to the ascorbic acid levels; 20% for tocopherol, 23% regarding vitamin A.

These results will be discussed and compared to the younger subjects (age 18–24). Conclusions concerning the use of blood-levels as indicators oft/nutrient intake for antioxidants will be drawn.

Use of probability calculations for predicting prevalence of iron deficiency among Danish women

J. HARALDSDÓTTIR

Research Department of Human Nutrition, The Royal Veterinary and Agricultural University, Copenhagen, Denmark

Today there is considerable theoretical interest in using probability calculations on dietary survey results for predicting the prevalence of nutrient deficiencies in a population[4]. However, there is a serious obstacle to the practical use of this approach: the limited knowledge of the nutrient requirements (on which the probability calculations are based).

One of the most studied nutrient requirements is the iron requirement of young women. For this nutrient both the mean and the basic distribution of the requirement have been described. Thus, if representative and valid iron intake data are available, there is a good basis for calculating the prevalence of iron deficiency among young women.

We have calculated the prevalence of iron deficiency among Danish women in fertile age, based on iron intake data from a nationwide dietary survey in 1985[1,2]. The calculated prevalences (e.g.: 11% in the age group 25–44 yrs.) compare reasonably well with the results of studies on iron status in Danish women, measured as serum ferritin[3].

This result indicates that the probability calculations are useful for predicting the prevalence of iron deficiency among young women. However, there are certain reservations to this conclusion: first of all the serum ferritin results are not necessarily representative of young Danish women in general, as they are based on small samples. Secondly, some of the assumptions included in our prevalence calculations may be questioned.

References

1 Haraldsdóttir J, Holm L, Jensen JH and Møller A. Danskernes kostvaner. 1985. 1. Hovedresultater. Levnedsmiddelstyrelsen, publ.nr.136, 1986. (With an English summary).
2 Haraldsdóttir J, Holm L, Jensen JH and Møller A. Danskernes kostvaner 1985. 2. Hvem spiser hvad? Levnedsmiddelstyrelsen, publ.nr.154, 1987.8 (With an English summary).
3 Milman N. (Unpublished results presented at the 4th Nordic nutrition conference, Odense, 1988).
4 Nutrient adequacy. Assessment using food consumption surveys. National% Academy Press, Washington DC, 1986.

Zinc protoporphyrin as a screening test for iron deficiency in children

M.B. DUGGAN and G. STEELS

Departments of Paediatrics & Haematology, University of Sheffield & Sheffield Childrens Hospital, Sheffield, United Kingdom

The prevalence of iron deficiency in British children is uncertain. Studies of British Asian children indicate a high prevalence of iron deficiency especially in the second year of life[1,2]. We studied iron status in 125 healthy Asian children aged between 4 and 40 months, and 40 white British children attending hospital. The serum ferritin, determined by immunoradiometry, was the reference method; the red cell zinc protoporphyrin (ZPP) was also determined by the protofluor method[3]. The performance of the ZPP as an index of iron deficiency was compared with that of the serum ferritin. The serum ferritin was low < 10mcg/1 in 47 children; and the ZPP was high > 80mcmol/mol Haem in 63 children. The prevalence of iron deficiency was estimated by the ZPP and serum ferritin respectively as 33,6% and 40% in Asian children and as 32.5% and 12.5% in white children in hospital.

The sensitivity of the ZPP as an indicator was 74% and 40% in healthy Asian and hospitalized white children respectively; the specificity was similar in the two groups 77% cf. 69%. The positive predictive value (PPV) of the ZPP as an index was 62% cf. 15% for healthy Asian and hospitalized white children respectively.

The possible influence of factors which might have resulted in false positive values for the ZPP or false negative values for the serum ferritin viz early infancy, and infection respectively was considered by further analyses from which data on infants and on infected children were separately excluded. These factors were considered to be of minor importance.

The significantly higher sensitivity and PPV of the ZPP in healthy Asian children is probably an effect of the difference in prevalence of iron deficiency between the two groups of children rather than an effect of confounding factors such as infection. The ZPP test which is easier and cheaper to perform than the serum ferritin is recommended as a screening test for groups at risk of iron deficiency.

References

1 Erhardt P. Br Med J 1986;292:90–93.
2 Grindulis H et al. Arch Dis Childhood 1986;61:843-848.
3 Labbe R et al. Meth Haematol 1980;44–58.

Serum ferritin: a biomarker of high iron intake in obese menstruating women

J. FRICKER and M. APFELBAUM

INSERM, Faculté Bichat, Paris, France

The study was carried out on 896 women. The subjects were distributed into three groups: 314 non obese (BMI < 27.3), 318 midly obese (27.3 < BMI < (32.3), 264 massively obese (BMI > 32.3).

Food intake was assessed with a dietary history questionnaire. Estimated energy intake varied significantly across corpulence groups: the greater the corpulence, the higher the energy intake. The relationship persisted after adjustment for age. Iron and protein intake were also significantly greater in obese. Does such an increase in iron intake lead to greater iron stores in obese women?

Twenty obese women and twenty non-obese control subjects matched for age and contraception were studied. Obese women consumed significantly more iron than did the non-obese women. Daily iron intake in the non-obese group was lower than the recommended dietary intake (RDI) of 15 mg in menstruating women whereas it was higher than the RDI in the obese group. The obese group showed significantly higher hemoglobin (137 ± 9 vs 129 ± 10g/l, x ± SD; $p < 0.01$), hematocrit (0.41 ± 0.02 vs 0.39 ± 0.03, $p < 0.05$) and serum ferritin concentrations (48.0 ± 44.3 vs 25.8 ± 19.5 mg/l, $p < 0.05$).

Thus, in obese women high iron intake are confirmed by high serum ferritin level. Obese women would appear to be a group at low risk of iron deficiency. However, this risk could be enhanced by the decrease in iron intake linked to the prescription of a low-calorie diet. On the other hand, systematic iron-fortification programs could enhance the prevalence of iron overload in these subjects.

Relationships among diet, urinary nitrogen excretion and growth of the elementary school children in urban and rural areas of Korea

H.Y. PAIK

Department of Food and Nutrition, Sookmyung Women's University, Seoul, Korea. Presently, Institute of Social Medicine, Free University of Berlin, Berlin, Germany

To understand the relationships among the dietary intake, urinary nitrogen (N) excretion, and growth of Korean children of 10–14 years of age, a nutritional survey was conducted in 38 children in Seoul and 36 children in a rural area of Korea. Food intake was recorded and 12-hour overnight urines were collected for the consecutive two days. Height (Ht) and weight (Wt) of each child were measured. Mean daily intakes of energy, carbohydrate, protein, animal protein, and fat were calculated from the food intake records. Urine samples were analyzed for total N and creatinine excretion. Height and weight of the children were compared to the standard values for Korean children for age and sex to calculate Ht-for-age and Wt-for-age. Mean values of the Ht-for-age and Wt-for-age of the children were 93.73 ± 3.82 and 79.20 ± 12.3 in the rural area and 97.79 ± 4.16 and 103.5 ± 20.2 in Seoul. The differences were significant ($p < 0.001$). Mean Wt-for-Ht were 96.21 ± 9.05 in the rural area and 110.4 ± 18.0 in Seoul ($p < 0.0001$). Distributions of Ht-for-age and Wt-for-age of the children in the two areas, according to the criteria by Waterlow, were significantly different ($X^2= 35.35$, $p < 0.001$). Children in Seoul consumed significantly more energy, protein, animal protein, and fat ($p < 0.0001$). Distributions of energy intake among carbohydrates protein:fat were 56:15:29 in Seoul and 76:12:12 in the rural area ($X^2= 10.41$, $p < 0.01$). Mean daily overnight excretions of total N and creatinine were 1.80 ± 1.03 g and 442 ± 215 mg in children in the rural area and 2.66 ± 1.38 g and 679 ± 252 mg in children in Seoul. The differences of the mean values were significant in both components ($p < 0.005$). Urinary N excretions were most significantly correlated to animal protein intakes ($p < 0.001$), but also correlated to the intakes of energy ($p < 0.05$), protein ($p < 0.01$), and fat ($p < 0.01$). Among the dietary and urinary factors, animal protein intake ($r=0.43$, $p < 0.001$) and creatinine excretion ($r=0.40$, $p < 0.001$) showed the highest correlation to Ht-for-age of the children; fat intake ($r=0.60$, $p < 0.0000$) and total N ($r=0.45$, $p < 0.001$) were the variables most highly correlated to Wt-for-age. The regression model for Ht-for-age improved significantly when creatinine excretion was added to the model with only animal protein intake as independent variable (adjusted R^2 values 24.5 and 17.2 respectively). Similarly, the best regression model for Wt-for-age included urinary total N excretion together with fat intake (adjusted R^2 values 43.1 and 35.3 respectively).

The use of individual biomarkers for improving and validating household salt consumption data

C. LECLERCQ , A. TURRINI, A. RAGUZZINI, E. CIALFA and A. FERRO-LUZZI

National Institute of Nutrition, Roma, Italy

A precise knowledge of national dietary salt consumption may be needed when setting up large-scale programmes which attempt to lower sodium intakes for the prevention of hypertension. Household surveys, often performed and for many purposes, provide information on salt use of large representative populations. However, these data lead to gross overestimation of sodium intakes, because salt is partially discarded in cooking water and in uneaten foods.

The aim of this study is to show that salt consumption data obtained in country-wide household surveys can be improved and validated by the use of individual biomarkers.

A national food survey was conducted by the National Institute of Nutrition in 1980–1984 on a sample of 10,000 households. The household consumption of all foods, including salt, was determined by two weighed inventories at 7 days interval, during which a daily record of all foods purchased was kept. Actual food consumption was corrected for meal participation of each household member to obtain the daily consumption per capita. The sodium content of table and cooking salt used was 2.8 ± 2.8 g p.c. (mean ± sd). The sodium derived from foods (either processed or unprocessed), calculated from the Italian tables of food composition, amounted to 2.4 ± 0.9 g p.c. True total sodium intake was individually assessed in 357 subjects with the use of two combined biological markers (urinary sodium and para-amino benzoic acid). It was 3.6 ± 1.3 g, in agreement with previous individual surveys conducted in Italy. Sodium intake from table and cooking salt – assessed with the lithium marker technique – was 1.6 ± 0.9 g.

The combination of this measure with the weighing of salt disappearance in the subjects' home allowed to calculate that 60% of all salt used (at the table and in cooking) was not ingested.

After correction for this loss, total sodium intake estimated in the household survey was 3.5 ± 1.7 g p.c., in agreement with the data obtained in the individual survey. In the literature it is suggested that only cooking salt is lost (76% discard). The application of this factor would have led to a 30% overestimate of sodium intakes in our household surveys. Specific data on salt losses occurring in the population under study may be assessed with biomarkers. Valid estimate of sodium intakes can then be derived from household surveys.

Development of biomarkers and elucidation of pathogenesis – the example of konzo, a newly identified nutritional myelopathy*

H. ROSLING and T. TYLLESKÄR

International Child Health Unit, University Hospital, Uppsala, Sweden

Konzo is a recently identified disease with acute onset of varying degree of permanent but not progressive spastic paraparesis. Dietary studies during konzo epidemics in rural populations in Mozambique, Tanzania and Zaire have revealed an association between konzo occurrence and a prolonged consumption of insufficiently processed cassava roots. These dietary situations were induced by food shortage. Cassave roots, a major staple in Africa, contain cyanogenic glycosides that must be removed before consumption by efficient processing. Dietary cyanide exposure was thus suggested as the cause of a metabolic insult to motorneurons resulting in konzo.

Ecological studies comparing konzo-affected and non-affected populations showed correlation between konzo and increased serum and urinary levels of thiocyanate, the most used marker of dietary cyanide exposure. However, in case-control studies during epidemics the thiocyanate levels were similar in affected as well as non-affected individuals.

A cassava dominated diet is low in proteins, especially sulphur aminoacids, that in the human body provides sulphur for enzymatic detoxification of cyanide to thiocyanate. Ecological studies also showed an association between konzo and decreased urinary levels of inorganic sulphate, a biomarker for sulphur intake. A combination of high cyanide and low sulphur intake decreasing the rate and/or changing the pattern of cyanide detoxification was then implicated as the cause of konzo.

In the body the first defense against cyanide is a rapid reversible binding to the methemoglobin in blood. Disappearance of cyanide from blood thereafter depends on the availability of sulphur for conversion to thiocyanate. Blood cyanide levels are therefore a good marker of the combined effect of high cyanide and low sulphur intakes. We therefore developed a new method that enables measurement of blood cyanide levels during epidemiological surveys.

In an ecological study design we have found higher blood cyanide levels in old konzo cases than in non-affected individuals from the same population in Zaire. This corresponds to the finding of a ten-fold higher incidence of aggravating attacks in the old cases compared to first attack in non-affected. We have also found that the three konzo cases that so far have been investigated within hours of onset had much higher blood cyanide compared to controls, whereas thiocyanate were equal in both groups. These findings indicate a causal effect of high cyanide and low sulphur intake. Data from dietary interviews strongly suggest that konzo results from about one months exposure to the above described diet. We therefore want a biomarker for several weeks of high cyanide and low sulphur intake. This may be a method for determination of the cyanolysed fraction of albumin or of some specific product from the reaction between body proteins and high levels of blood cyanide.

Recent advances in neuroscience in fact suggest that the reaction products between cyanide and body proteins may act as an excitatory aminoacid and be the neurotoxic factor in konzo. We conclude that improvements of biomarkers run parallel to increased understanding of pathogenesis and vice versa. With the use of biomarkers epidemiology can go beyond identification of risk factors and be used for elucidation of pathogenesis.

*Konzo is the name of the paralysis in the language of the first affected population in Zaire.

List of participants

Page numbers, for contributions published in this book, are given in parentheses.

Australia

1 Truswell, A

Austria

2 Godina-Zarfl B, Wien
3 Maierhofer A, Pezud

Belgium

4 Guillaume M, Brussels
5 Schmitt A, Brussels

Denmark

6 Ewertz M, Copenhagen
7 Haraldsdottir J, Copenhagen (129)
8 Helsing E, Copenhagen
9 Larsen L, Brabrand
10 Michaelsen K, Frederiksberg
11 Overvad K, Aarhus
12 Tjønneland A, Copenhagen

Finland

13 Ahola I, Helsinki (103)
14 Alfthan G, Helsinki (106, 110, 112)
15 Aro A, Helsinki (103, 110, 112)
16 Hemminki K, Helsinki (59)
17 Huttunen J, Helsinki (110, 112)
18 Järvinen R, Kuopio (127)
19 Järvisalo J, Turku (123)
20 Tikkanen M, Helsinki (67)
21 Valsta L, Helsinki (90, 103)

France

22 Antoine J, Paris

23 Fricker J, Paris (131)
24 Rolland-Cachera M, Le Vésiner

Germany
25 Boeing H, Heidelberg (116)
26 Kersting M, Dortmund (82)
27 Kohlmeier-Arab L, Berlin (15, 128)
28 Melchert H, Berlin (95)
29 Pheifer-Zaek, Heidelberg
30 Stender M, Neuherberg
31 Thamm M, Berlin (128)

Indonesia
32 Rumawas J, Jakarta

Republic of Ireland
33 Cunningham K, Dublin

Israel
34 Kark J, Jerusalem (101)

Italy
35 Fidanza F, Perugia
36 La Vecchia C, Milan
37 Leclercq C, Roma
38 Scaccini C, Roma (98)
39 Turrini A, Roma

Korea
40 Paik H, Seoul (132)

Malta
41 Beluzzi M, Floriana

Norway
42 Drevon C, Oslo (93)
43 Johansson L, Oslo
44 Meltzer H, Oslo (111)
45 Nes M, Oslo

Portugal
46 Lopes Elias M, Torres Vedras

Spain
47 Barrenetxea M, Vitoria
48 Gómez Aracena J, Malaga (100)

49 Gomez Henry J, Sevilla
50 Mendez Martinez C, Sevilla
51 Pinedo Sanchez A, Malaga (100)

Sweden
52 Arvidsson-Lenner R, Göteborg
53 Elmstohl S, Malmö
54 Hallmans G, Umeâ
55 Hultén B, Göteborg
56 Johansson I, Umeâ
57 Karlström B, Uppsala
58 Rosling H, Uppsala (135)
59 Samuelson G, Trouhättan
60 Vessby B, Uppsala

Switzerland
61 Gey F, Bern (121)
62 Haller J, Basel

The Netherlands
63 Al M, Maastricht
64 Bausch-Goldbohm S, Zeist (118)
65 Beresteyn, van E, Ede
66 Berg van den H, Zeist
67 Blom J, Maarssen
68 Brandt van den P, Maastricht (118)
69 Breejen den H, Rotterdam
70 Drongelen van M, Maastricht
71 Duyn van C, Rotterdam
72 Faassen van D, Hulsberg (113)
73 Feskens E, Bilthoven
74 Feunekes G, Wageningen
75 Goeij de J, Delft (115)
76 Govers M, Ede
77 Grobbee D, Rotterdam
78 Groot de L, Wageningen (26)
79 Hermus R, Zeist (118)
80 Hertog M, Wageningen
81 Hiddink G, Maarssen
82 Hoffmans M, Bilthoven
83 Hofman Z, Zoetermeer
84 Hulshof K, Zeist
85 Hulshof T, Wageningen
86 Jacobs N, Leiden
87 Kampman E, Zeist
88 Kardinaal A, Zeist

89 Katan M, Wageningen (4)
90 Kempen K, Maastricht
91 Koe de W, Rijswijk
92 Kok F, Zeist (7, 27)
93 Kooy van der K, Wageningen
94 Kromhout D, Bilthoven
95 Leenen R, Wageningen
96 Leezer-de Hoog H, Zeist
97 Ocké M, Bilthoven
98 Ockhuizen T, Zeist
99 Pastoor F, Utrecht
100 Poppel van G, Zeist
101 Roodenburg A, Wageningen
102 Schouten E, Wageningen
103 Seidell J, Wageningen (102)
104 Spaaij C, Wageningen
105 Veer van 't P, Zeist (27, 106, 118)
106 Verboeket W, Maastricht
107 Verhagen H, Zeist
108 Vet de H, Maastricht
109 Vliet van T, Zeist
110 Voorrips L, Wageningen
111 Vrijer de F, Zeist
112 Westerterp K, Maastricht (76, 87)
113 Weusten M, Wageningen
114 Wielen van der R, Wageningen
115 Witteman J, Rotterdam
116 Zock P, Wageningen

United Kingdom
117 Albert C, London
118 Bingham S, Cambridge (41, 76, 78)
119 Black A, Cambridge (78, 80, 84)
120 Brunner E, London
121 Dagnelie P, London (96)
122 Duggan M, Sheffield (130)
123 Forman D, Oxford (53)
124 Livingstone M, Coleraine (78, 80)
125 Preunglampoo S, Southampton
126 Riemersma R, Edinburgh (90)
127 Rona R, London
128 Shortt C, Aberdeen
129 Strain S, Coleraine (80, 121)

USA
130 Crawford L, Albany

131 Kretsch M, San Francisco
132 Willett W, Boston (9)

USSR
133 Mazayev V, Moscow

Yugoslavia
134 Adamic M, Ljubljana